Principles of IMMUNODIAGNOSTICS

Principles of IMMUNODIAGNOSTICS

RALPH MICHAEL ALOISI, D.A. MT(ASCP)

Medical Technology Program Director,
Assistant Professor Biology and Chemistry,
University of Hartford,
West Hartford, Connecticut

with **148** illustrations

The C. V. Mosby Company

ST. LOUIS • TORONTO • LONDON 1979

Printed in the United States of America

The C. V. Mosby Company
11830 Westline Industrial Drive, St. Louis, Missouri 63141

Library of Congress Cataloging in Publication Data

Aloisi, Ralph Michael, 1945-
Principles of immunodiagnostics.

Bibliography: p.
Includes index.
1. Immunodiagnosis. I. Title.
RB46.5.A46 616.07'56 78-24471
ISBN 0-8016-0118-5

GW/M/M 9 8 7 6 5 4 3 2 1 01/D/050

To my wife

CAROL

for her unending patience and assistance

Preface

For decades, the specific and sensitive reaction of antigen with antibody has been utilized clinically as a diagnostic aid for the patient with infectious diseases. As researchers explored this miraculous reaction, it became evident that a powerful analytical tool was at hand. During the last decade, clinical tests based on the immune reaction have grown at a phenomenal rate. No longer is serology hidden in dark, crowded corners of the clinical microbiology laboratory. A new discipline of laboratory medicine is rapidly passing from infancy to adolescence. In most major laboratories this departmental section is designated "Immunodiagnostics" or "Clinical Immunology." This analytical laboratory traverses the classical boundaries within the department of pathology and is currently utilized in research, diagnostics, and for the management of patients with a wide variety of disorders.

Currently available immunology books fall into several categories: the research-oriented techniques books, the encyclopedia volumes of procedures books, the comprehensive immunology texts, and references on immunopathology. The time has come for a book to deal with the basic principles of immunochemistry applied to the diagnostic field. The purpose is not to provide step-by-step procedures but rather to isolate and lay down fundamental concepts. This book attempts to provide a logical and relevant approach to this most fascinating field. The major objective is to elucidate and apply basic concepts so that the student of laboratory medicine can better deal with the magic of the immunoassay kits that now flood the marketplace. Clearly, a thorough understanding of fundamental principles provides the laboratorian with a means for keeping abreast of new assays and better controlling and understanding of the classical immunologic tests.

The text is divided into two major sections. The first section isolates fundamental concepts of protein chemistry and immunology. Those characteristics that govern protein behavior are discussed to provide better understanding of antibody activity. The immunology reviewed in this section is that portion of this immense field that is necessary to understand clinical applications. Section two of the text classifies and categorizes a selection of currently used immunodiagnostic techniques. The generalizations developed are applicable to both present and future immunoassays. The clinical procedures reviewed not only provide interest and relevancy but are critical examples of the category of tests. Clinical examples briefly describe the principle, methodology, interferences, clinical correlations, and interpretations. At the end of each chapter "Readings and Resources" direct the student, instructor, and laboratorian to current and classical procedure references.

While not primarily designed to be a reference book, this text aids in the interpretation of tests, in the choice of methodologies, and in developing quality control techniques as well as identifying common pitfalls or sources of error. The primary audience for this book is the student of laboratory medicine who wishes to better utilize the powerful analytical capabilities of immunologic tests. No attempt is made to review the rapidly expanding area of cellular immunology and its clinical applications, for this area is beyond the scope and "basic" premise of this text.

The diligent and systematic research of scientists, such as Berson and Yallow, has provided modern medicine with techniques of immense value. It is the clinical laboratorian who must make valid use of these analytical techniques.

I wish to thank Drs. M. Sochard, G. Roberts, and E. Kennedy for their guidance. Dr. Eleanor Griffith offered helpful suggestions in her review of portions of the manuscript. The contributions by Millipore Biomedica, Hyland Laboratories, Kallestad Laboratories, Ames Company, and Helena Laboratories were extremely helpful. The credit for converting the handwritten manuscript to legible text goes to the fine secretarial assistance of Debra Becker. Finally, I wish to thank my family for their patience and encouragement during this endeavor.

Ralph Michael Aloisi

Contents

SECTION ONE

FUNDAMENTAL CONCEPTS

The clinical laboratory practitioner must be aware of the factors that may influence an assay. A review of the basic concepts of protein chemistry as well as the modern tenets of immunology is a necessary requisite to a complete understanding of the fundamental principles of immunodiagnostics. The clinical laboratorian must be prepared to maximally utilize the powerful tools of modern clinical immunochemistry. This section includes protein structure and function, immunoglobulins, antigens and antigenicity, and the interaction of antigen-antibody.

CHAPTER 1

Proteins

Proteins are the expression of DNA and one of the products of evolution. These molecules are physiologically active and perform a variety of functions. The term "operational molecule" has been used to describe the biologically specific function of proteins. Proteins are most frequently classified structurally. A classification based on the common functional characteristic, specific binding of molecules or ligands, helps emphasize the operational nature of proteins. The common functional characteristic of the proteins in Table 1 is recognition and specific binding of other molecules. What is it that enables proteins such as enzymes and antibodies to specifically bind their appropriate ligands, substrates, and antigens? Clearly, ligand binding is the common denominator. A review of those factors involved in binding in reality is a review of protein interaction. An understanding of protein interactions provides insight into the binding of all ligands by these operational molecules.

What is it that determines binding activity of proteins? Enzymes are catalytic proteins with readily measurable activity. The reaction of enzyme with substrate produces a decrease in substrate and an increase in product. Simultaneous advances in instrumentation and in enzymology have made enzymes excellent models for the study of protein structure and function. Christian Anfinsen carefully studied the activity of the enzyme ribonuclease in an altered and native

Table 1. Functional classification of proteins

Type	Function	Type example
I	Catalytic	Enzymes
II	Immune	Antibodies
III	Transport	Ceruloplasmin
IV	Regulatory	Insulin
V	Contractive	Myosin

state. The term "native state" refers to the three-dimensional shape the enzyme would have in its natural physiologic environment. In the altered state ribonuclease lost activity (denaturation). If the altered molecule was exposed to certain conditions, it would twist, bend, and fold until it regained its natural shape or conformation. As the enzyme regained its native state, it regained its activity (renaturation). One hypothesis to account for this phenomenon is that the primary structure (the sequence of amino acids) dictates the final conformation of the protein molecule. Anfinsen's study is similar to the following somewhat bizarre hypothetical experiment. A finely tooled Swiss watch is taken apart and the pieces placed in a bag. The bag is shaken. Given enough time, the watch parts would find their proper positions and the watch would resume its shape and finally its activity. There is something more than reality in this animated hypothetical study, but it does serve to clarify Anfinson's problem. It is now known that structure dictates function! Is it the fine chemical detail of molecules or the gross shape that determines specificity and activity? What energy is used to drive his altered enzyme to its native state? The concepts involved are fundamental to molecular biology and indeed to any form of protein chemistry such as enzymology or immunology.

PROTEIN CHEMISTRY

Amino acid bondings and interactions

Most proteins when treated with acids, bases, or proteolytic enzymes are degraded to alpha amino acids. The approximately 20 amino acids usually derived from this hydrolytic process all have a similar core structure and differ primarily by their side groups or R-groups (Fig. 1-1). The varied structure of R-groups provides each amino acid core with a differing chemical behavior. The in vitro combination of amino acids to form chains occurs via a condensation process with the exclusion of water (Fig. 1-2).

The in vivo process is by far more complex but the end product is the same, a linear molecule of polyamino acid. When this polyamino acid reaches a length of 40 amino acids, it is considered, by some, to be a protein. The line between polyamino acid and protein is arbitrary and frequently disputed. The peptide bonds formed between the amino acids account for the use of the term "polypeptide" as a synonym for polyamino acid.

Peptide bond. The peptide bond, seen in Fig. 1-2, is formed between the amino group of one amino acid and the carboxyl group of another amino acid. The peptide bond, referred to by some scientists as an amide bond, has a resonating character (Fig. 1-3). The bond between the carbon and nitrogen would be expected to have a bond length of 1.49 Å, but due to the partial double-bonded nature of this bond, the actual length is 1.32 Å. The resonance on the peptide bond gives it some rigid features and partially limits its free rotation. The rigid or planar features of the peptide bond alternating with bonds that contain free rotation would tend to allow the molecule to fall into a randomly coiling conformation. As

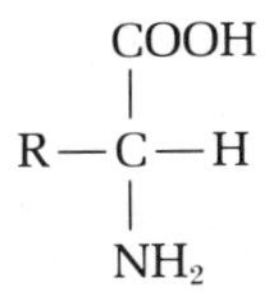

Fig. 1-1. Typical alpha-amino acid demonstrating common core and site for variations in side group or R-group attachment.

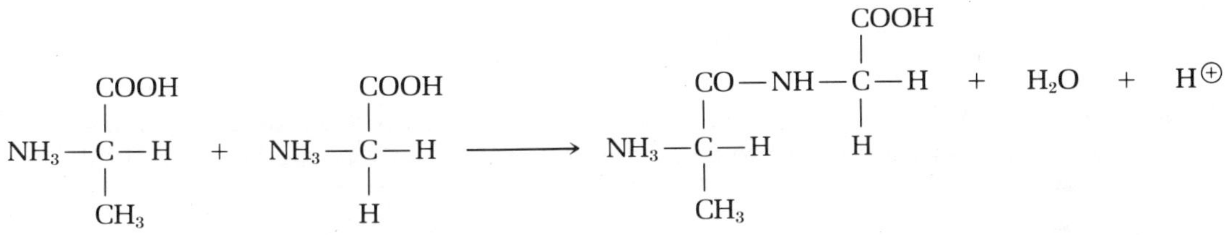

Fig. 1-2. Condensation reaction of first amino acid, alanine, with second amino acid, glycine, results in formation of alanylglycine. Formation of a two-amino acid chain is the result of peptide-bond formation and water exclusion.

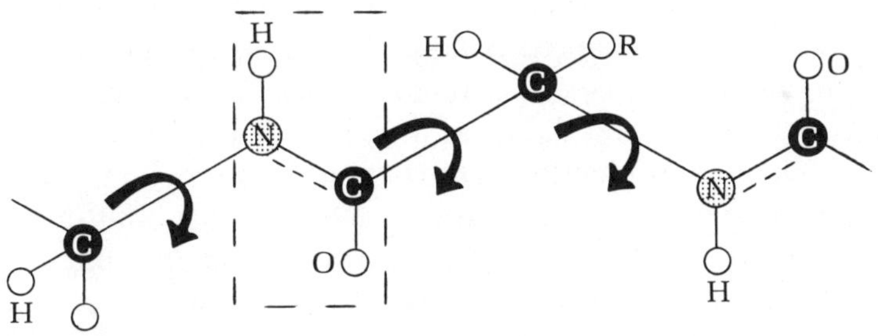

Fig. 1-3. Segment of protein molecule. Arrows indicate bonds with free rotation and dotted enclosures indicate peptide bonds. Note free rotation does not exist at the peptide bond.

the molecule begins to take on this randomly coiling shape, the amino acids within the structure apply restrictions on the developing structure. For example, an amino acid with an enormous bulky side group could inhibit this coiling by competing for available space. This type of interference is referred to as steric hindrance. A variety of forces such as intrachain bonding can thrust the molecule into its final shape. Therefore peptide bonds and steric hindrance can effect the interactions of amino acids and the conformation of proteins. However, there are other significant interactions that affect amino acid bonding and protein conformation.

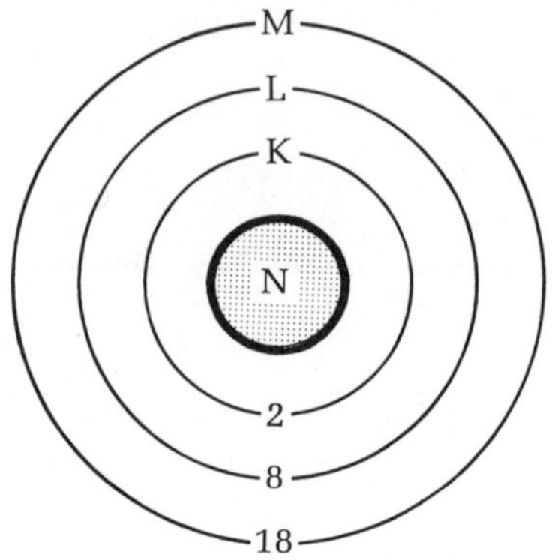

Fig. 1-4. Diagrammatic representation of an atom showing two electrons are required to fill K orbit, eight are required to fill L orbit, and eighteen are needed to fill M orbit.

Ionic bonding. Stability is the final goal of every atom and molecule. We are well aware of the decay of radioactive isotopes. Decay is a means for the isotope to become a stable molecule. A fundamental concept in chemistry is that the filling of electron orbits tends to yield inertness or stability. Fig. 1-4 shows the number of electrons required to fill the K, L, and M orbits of any atom.

The greater the distance from the outermost orbiting, negatively charged electrons to the positively charged nucleus, the more readily that electron can be removed. An atom with one electron in its M orbit can be considered to have a low ionization potential, and therefore little energy is required to remove that electron. An atom such as chloride has seven electrons in its L orbit; this atom would be more apt to gain one electron in order to fill that orbit than to loose its seven outer electrons. Chloride has a high ionization potential and a high affinity for electrons. Electron transfer will occur when an atom with a low ionization potential comes into proximity of an atom with a high electron affinity. The transfer of the outermost electron of sodium to chloride leaves both atoms oppositely charged. The positively charged sodium ion will now be attracted to the negatively charged chloride ion. The formation of an ionic bond, actually an interaction or an electrostatic force, leaves a net charge of zero. Any marked increase in the free ion concentration in the solution that contains the sodium and chloride ions would reduce the probability of bonding between the sodium ion and the chloride ion.

Covalent bond. In ionic bonding the key concept was the complete transfer of an electron. In covalent bonding the crucial point is an incomplete electron transfer. Covalent bonds are incomplete transfers of electrons between two or more atoms. Hydrogen has a high ionization potential and a high electron affinity. The reaction of one hydrogen atom with another hydrogen atom can occur by sharing each others' one electron. This sharing process acts to fill the K orbit of both atoms (Fig. 1-5).

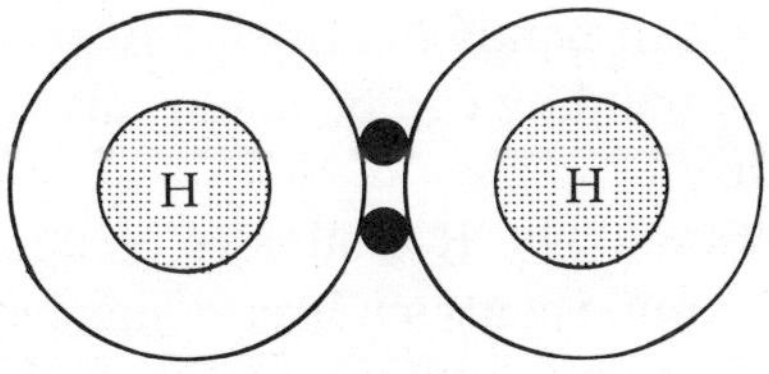

Fig. 1-5. Hydrogen gas; hydrogen atoms are covalently linked. Each atom shares the other one's electron.

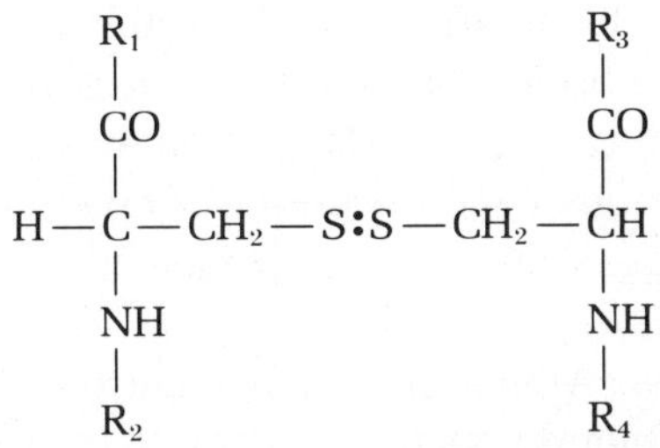

Fig. 1-6. Cysteine residues on two separate polypeptide chains covalently bonded to form cystine.

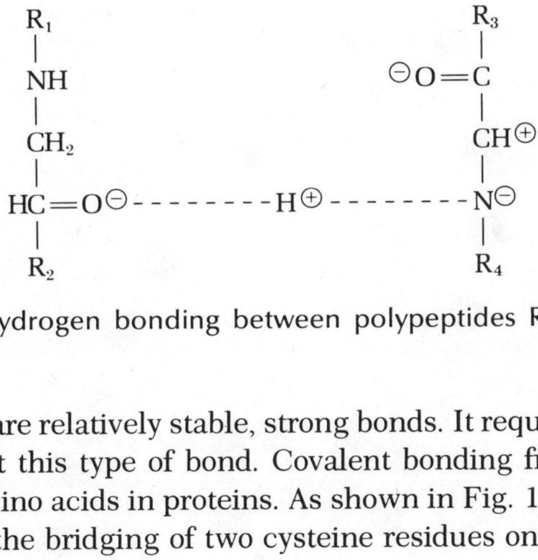

Fig. 1-7. Interchain hydrogen bonding between polypeptides R_1 to R_2 and R_3 to R_4.

Covalent bonds are relatively stable, strong bonds. It requires extremely harsh treatment to disrupt this type of bond. Covalent bonding frequently occurs between particular amino acids in proteins. As shown in Fig. 1-6, this type of bonding can be seen in the bridging of two cysteine residues on two separate chains to form cystine.

Hydrogen bond. The hydrogen atom tends to share its electron with other atoms, hence it is predominantly a positively charged proton. As such, the hydrogen may be mutually attracted by negatively charged atoms or ions. Under certain circumstances, hydrogen can find itself suspended between two negatively charged ions, forming the hydrogen bond. As shown in Fig. 1-7, hydrogen bonding frequently occurs between polypeptide chains but can also occur within a single chain (intrachain). Although each hydrogen bond is relatively weak, the great number of hydrogen bonds in any one molecule can add up to a substantial effect. This type of bonding can be readily altered by pH changes and/or changes in ionic strength.

Hydrophobic interactions. The R-groups of certain amino acids are hydrophobic or "water-hating." Amino acids such as valine, leucine, and phenylalanine are hydrophobic, and these amino acids are unable to form hydrogen bonds with water. Hydrophobic amino acids are electrically neutral; their positive and negative centers coincide, hence they are referred to as nonpolar. The lack of polarity on these amino acids is responsible for their inability to hydrogen bond with water. Hydrophobic amino acids in an aqueous solution are driven together as are oil droplets on water. Hydrophobic interaction often is the driving force that folds and bends polypeptides, forming globular proteins excluding water. As shown in Fig. 1-8, hydrophobic amino acids form nucleation sites or points of folding, and hydrophilic amino acids are driven to the surface of the molecule to interact with water.

Van der Waals forces. Atoms and their electron clouds interact with other atoms and their electron clouds. As the two atoms approach each other, the electron cloud of one is attracted to the nucleus of the other. At a certain critical dis-

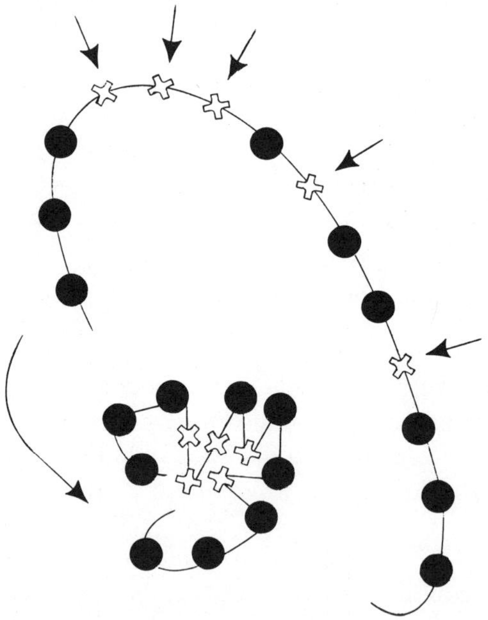

Fig. 1-8. Polar amino acids that readily interact with water (hydrophilic) are indicated by —●—. Nonpolar (hydrophobic) amino acids are indicated by —✲—. Note that polypeptide tends to form nucleation sites at nonpolar amino acid, resulting in conformation that allows hydrophilic amino acids to remain at surface of molecule.

tance, as the two atoms approach each other, the clouds repel each other. The actual force can be mathematically derived. Van der Waals interactions are nonspecific and are a measure of attraction and repulsion of any two atoms. The strength and direction of this force are critically dependent on distance.

Amino acid chemistry

Classification of amino acids. Each amino acid has unique physical and chemical characteristics. Classifying amino acids by their polarity provides a functional approach to amino acids and a more useful approach to protein structure and function (note Tables 2 to 4).

Acid-base properties of amino acids. All amino acids have at least two ionizable groups ($R—NH_3^+$ and R—COOH). Like other weak acids, amino acids do not completely dissociate. The term "protonic equilibria" refers to the association and dissociation of proton donors and proton acceptors. In solution this equilibria can be expressed as seen in equations 1-1 and 1-2.

$$R—COOH \rightleftharpoons RCOO^- + H^+ \qquad \textbf{(Eq. 1-1)}$$

$$R—NH_3^+ \rightleftharpoons H^+ + R—NH_2 \qquad \textbf{(Eq. 1-2)}$$

The R—COOH and $R—NH_3^+$ are both acid groups capable of donating a hydrogen ion. The $R—COO^-$ and $R—NH_2$ groups are the conjugate bases of the above weak acids. The R—COOH is a far better acid than the $R—NH_3^+$ group. At a pH of 6.0 to 7.0 R—COOH readily donates its hydrogen ion. Even at a pH as low as 4 the R—COOH group may donate its hydrogen ion. $R—NH_3^+$ tends not to give up its hydrogen ion or proton below a pH of 9.0. As is seen in Tables 2 to 4, each amino acid group has slightly varying pK values. pK is the negative log of the dissociation constant; the larger the dissociation constant, the smaller the pK and the stronger the acid. The pK of an amino or carboxyl group is the pH at which 50% of these groups would be dissociated and 50% would be associated.

Although most students are put on the defensive at the sight of pH, pK, and pI, it is important to understand the implications in their use. For example, if we were to look at glycine, the pK of R—COOH group is 2.34, the pK_2 of $R—NH_3^+$ is 9.6. At a pH of 2.34, 50% of the R—COOH would be protonated and 50% dissociated. At a pH of 9.6, 50% of $R—NH_3^+$ groups would be protonated and 50% dissociated. As can be seen in Fig. 1-9, glycine at a physiologic pH of 6 to 7 is partially protonated and partially dissociated.

The isoelectric point (pI) of an amino acid is that pH where the net charge per amino acid is equal to zero. With a net charge of zero, amino acids or proteins are at their pI and would not migrate in an electric field. For a diprotonic molecule such as glycine the pI would be calculated using equation 1-3.

$$pI = \frac{pK_1 + pK_2}{2} \qquad \textbf{(Eq. 1-3)}$$

Table 2. Hydrophobic amino acids with nonpolar R-groups

Amino acid	Three-letter code	One-letter code	R-group	R—COOH pK	R—NH_3^+ pK₂
Alanine	Ala	A	CH_3	2.34	9.69
Valine	Val	V	CH_3 \ CH_2— / CH_3	2.32	9.62
Leucine	Leu	L	CH_3 \ CH—CH_2— / CH_3	2.36	9.60
Isoleucine	Ile	I	CH_3—CH_2 \ CH— / CH_3	2.36	9.68
Phenylalanine	Phe	F	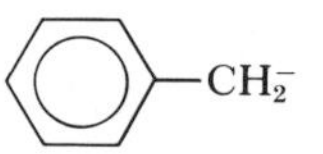	1.83	9.13
Proline	Pro	P	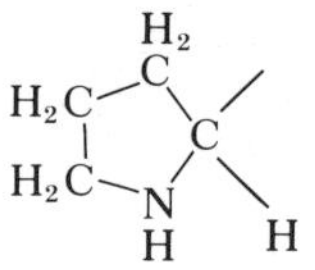	1.99	10.60
Tryptophan	Trp	W	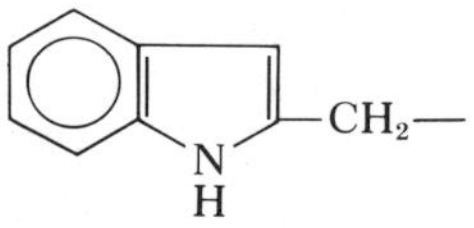	2.38	9.39
Methionine	Met	M	CH_3—S—CH_2—CH_2—	2.28	9.73

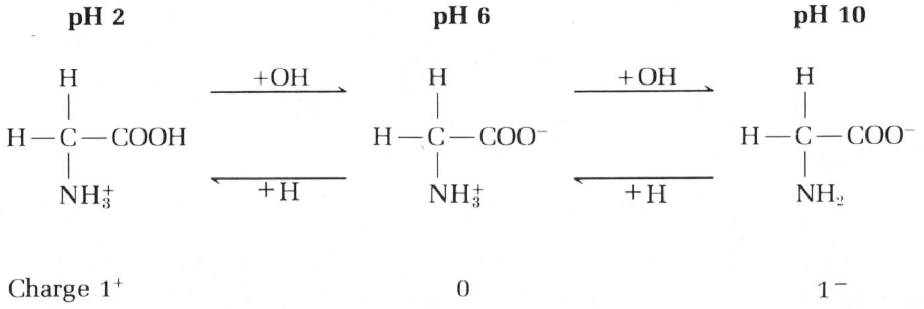

Fig. 1-9. pH titration of amino acid glycine showing ionization and charge distribution at varied pH ranges.

Table 3. Amino acids with more soluble polar R-group

Amino acid	Three-letter symbol	One-letter symbol	R-group	pK R—COOH	pK_2 R—NH_3^+
Glycine	Gly	G	H	2.34	9.60
Serine	Ser	S	$HO-CH_2-$	2.21	9.15
Threonine	Thr	T	$CH_3-CH(OH)-$	2.63	10.43
Cysteine	Cys	C	$HS-CH_2-$	1.71	10.78
Tyrosine	Tyr	Y	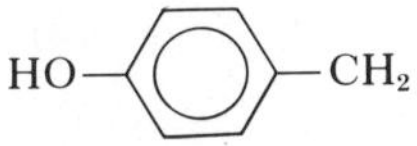	2.20	9.11
Aspargenine	Asn	N	$NH_2-C(=O)-CH_2-$		
Glutamine	Gln	Q	$NH_2-C(=O)-CH_2-CH_2-CH_2-$	2.17	9.13

Table 4. Amino acid with a net positively charged R-group in the physiologic pH range

Amino acid	Three-letter symbol	One-letter symbol	R-group	pK R—COOH	pK_2 R—NH_3^+
Lysine	Lys	L	$H_2-N-C-(CH_2)_3-$	2.18	8.95
Arginine	Arg	R	$H_2N-C(=NH)-(CH_2)_3-$	2.17	9.04
Histidine	His	H	$HC{=}CH-CH_2-$ (ring: HC=CH, HN, NH, C; +)	1.82	9.70

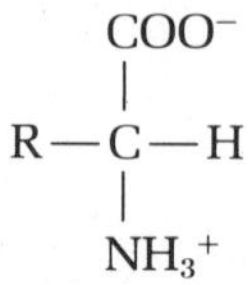

Fig. 1-10. Zwitterion form of certain amino acids at pH range of 6 to 7. Note balanced charge distribution.

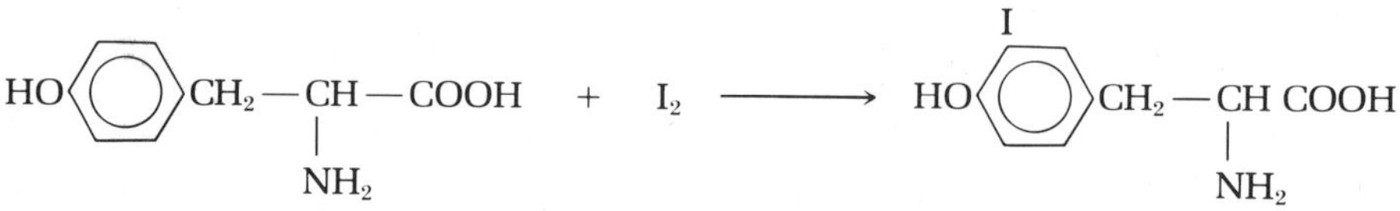

Fig. 1-11. Reaction of iodine with amino acid tyrosine.

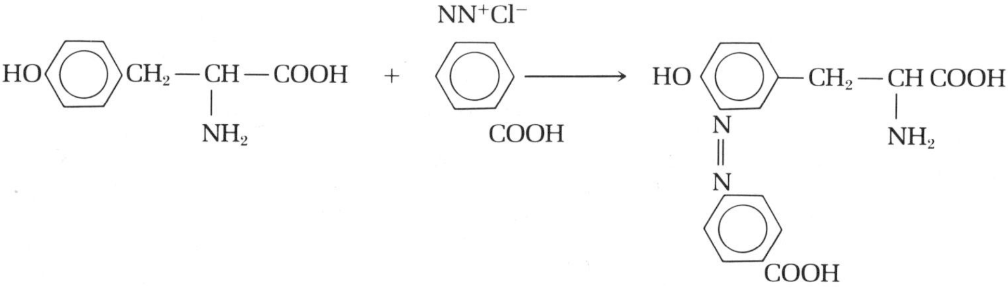

Fig. 1-12. Reaction of diazo salts with tyrosine.

The neutral amino acid (Fig. 1-10) with equal positive and negative charges is referred to as a "zwitterion." This amino acid form is the type most likely to exist at physiologic pH's, which are near the pI of the amino acid.

Significant chemical reactions of amino acids. Saturated hydrocarbon R-group amino acids, those without double bonds such as glycine, valine, leucine, alanine, and isoleucine, are stable and relatively inert. These amino acids primarily interact via hydrogen bonding and hydrophobic and Van der Waals forces.

Serine and threonine are hydroxyl R-group amino acids. Phosphoric acid and polysaccharides are often attached through these amino acids, producing phosphoproteins and glycoproteins. The hydroxyl group is frequently available for hydrogen bonding. Tyrosine, tryptophan, and phenylalanine are aromatic amino acids that strongly absorb ultraviolet light at 277 nanometers (nm). As shown in Fig. 1-11, tyrosine is often the point of attachment for iodine and its isotopes. Diazo salts (Fig. 1-12) can be readily added to tyrosine. Lysine, arginine, and histidine are positively charged basic amino acids with extra amino groups (at pH 7). The additional amino groups are free to ionize and can be involved in several reactions. If the alpha amino group is involved in a peptide linkage, the epsilon

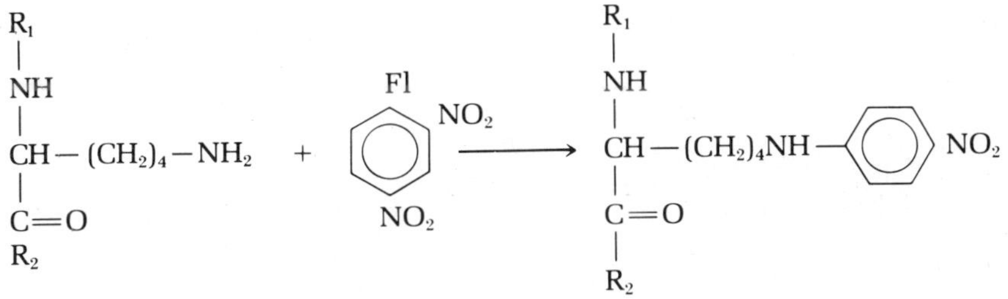

Fig. 1-13. Addition of difluorobenzene to amino groups of lysine, within polypeptide chain, R_1 to R_2.

amino group can be used for the addition of aromatic nitro compounds to proteins. Additions, such as that shown in Fig. 1-13, are often used to attach fluorescent molecules to protein. Fluorescent molecules are molecules that emit a precise wavelength of light when excited with a particular ultraviolet light.

In summary, all amino acids have a similar central core structure and all are involved in acid-base equilibria, but even with these common features they remain distinctly different. Although the sequential linear arrangement of amino acids is determined by the DNA code and is modified through evolution, the uniqueness of each amino acid is due to the particular characteristics of their R-groups.

PROTEIN STRUCTURE

DNA dictates amino acid sequence but what governs protein conformation and what factors determine shape? Does a newly formed polypeptide or protein mold into any shape, or is this determined in advance? What forces dictate conformation? The relationship of one amino acid to its neighbor is called the primary structure. DNA determines the primary structure. When amino acid number one is linked to amino acid number two, their unique chemical and physical characteristics begin to interact. After the addition of amino acid number three, the side chain may be attracted to the side chains of amino acid one and two or it may be repelled by the other amino acid side chains. In order that the structure reach its most stable conformation in an aqueous medium, polar amino acids attempt to maximize hydrogen bonding. The planar rigidity of the peptide bond tends to force a linear molecule into a circular staircase (a helix). This helical structure (Fig. 1-14) brings amino acids (short distances apart) together and allows greater hydrogen bonding.

Amino acids, such as hydroxyproline and proline with their heterocyclic cores, disrupt alpha helix formation by interfering with the planar peptide bond. The alpha helix is an example of a secondary structure and describes the interactions of nearby amino acids. As predicted by "protonic equilibria," pH changes cause alterations in ionization of R-groups, carboxyl groups, and amino groups.

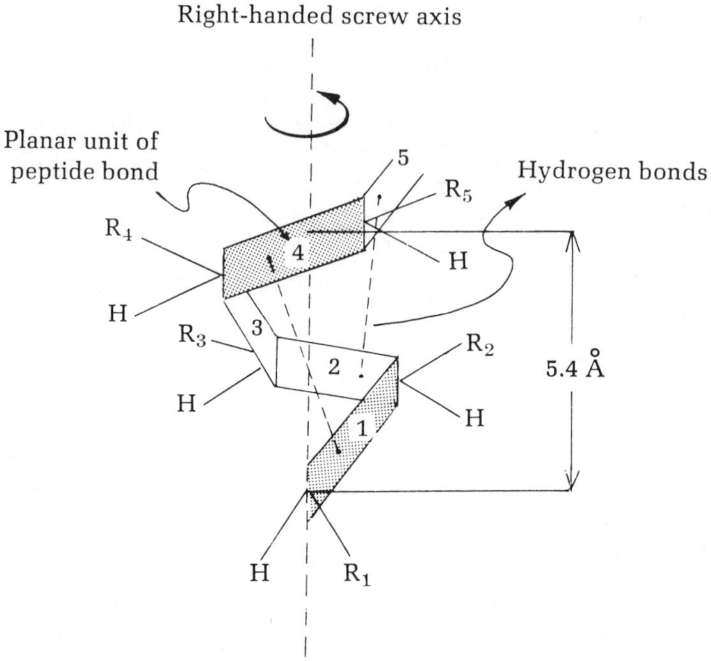

Fig. 1-14. Alpha helix is example of secondary structure and demonstrates interaction of nearby amino acids. Note intrachain hydrogen bonding. (From Montgomery, R., et al.: Biochemistry: a case oriented approach, ed. 2, St. Louis, 1977, The C. V. Mosby Co.)

Modification of pH can cause changes in secondary structure. Glutamic acid, for example, at a low pH has no charge; its carboxyl R-group would have little effect on structure if it were in an alpha helical area of a polypeptide. If the pH were raised sharply, glutamic acid would take on a minus two charge. The now negatively charged glutamic acid would repel other negatively charged amino acids and therefore would act as a so-called helix breaker. Lysine, with its epsilon amino group, would have no charge at high pH values but would have a positive charge at a low pH. Lysine would act as a helix breaker at low pH values and would tend to induce random coiling. Bulky R-groups of amino acids such as isoleucine may sterically inhibit alpha helix formation. As demonstrated in Fig. 1-15, hydrogen bonding between two polypeptide chains can produce what is known as the beta structure or the pleated sheet. Most proteins, in their natural conformation, contain pleated sheet, alpha helix, and random coil areas.

After the primary and secondary structure is established other forces begin to change the protein conformation. Hydrophobic R-groups may be driven together to form a nucleation site. This nucleation site is a point that may initiate folding of the polypeptide. When the polypeptide has completed folding and bending, the end product contains polar amino acids on the surface. These polar amino acids increase solubility by allowing hydrogen bonding with water.

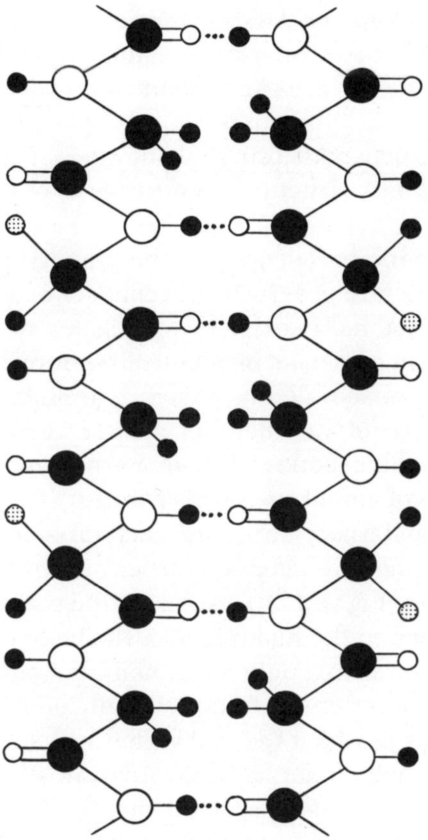

Fig. 1-15. Beta pleated sheet with interchain hydrogen bonding.

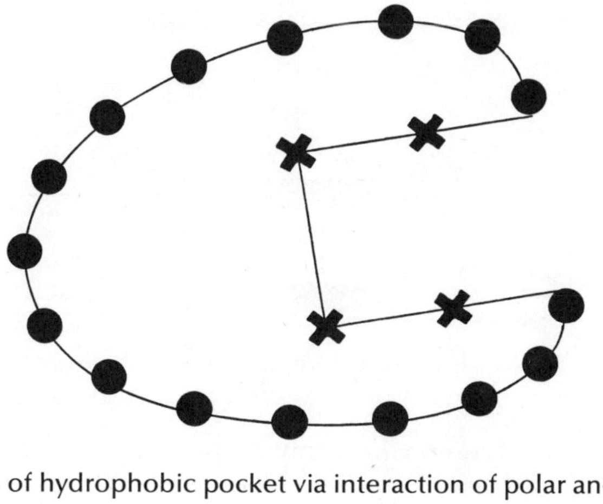

Fig. 1-16. Formation of hydrophobic pocket via interaction of polar and nonpolar amino acids.

Through interactions of Van der Waals forces, electrostatic forces, and hydrogen bonding, the polypeptide takes on a more stable orientation. A string of hydrophobic amino acids at the surface of a protein can produce a hydrophobic pocket (Fig. 1-16).

The folding of the polypeptide brings about interaction of distant amino acids and is known as the tertiary structure. In retrospect we can now make the statements that:

1. DNA dictates amino acid sequence, the primary structure.
2. The primary structure governs the secondary and tertiary structures.

Many proteins, if not most, exist in aggregates of subunits. Hemoglobin and antibody both exist as a pair of identical subunits. Hemoglobin consists of four protein chains noncovalently linked, two alpha and two beta chains. Immunoglobulins consist of variations of a basic protein chain structure covalently linked by disulfide bonds. The quaternary structure of proteins describes the interactions of amino acids on separate polypeptide chains. All known forces play a role in quaternary structure, including covalent bonding. An example of covalent bonding in quaternary structure can be seen in the immunoglobulin of the IgG class (Fig. 1-17). Cysteine at the carboxyl end of a light chain dimerizes with a cysteine in the mid region of the heavy chains on an IgG molecule. If the heavy chain was in a tight alpha helix, it would be likely that the secondary structure would interfere with the covalent bonding of cysteines. To overcome this, evolution has provided the mid region with high proline and hydroxyl proline concentrations, which act as helix breakers. The IgG example emphasizes the importance of amino acid sequence to final structure.

The existence of this protein in its native conformation is clearly governed by many factors. The major influence, however, is the primary structure. This protein is in a precarious state for its activities are dependent on its conformation and the conformation is dependent on the combined effect of many weak bonds.

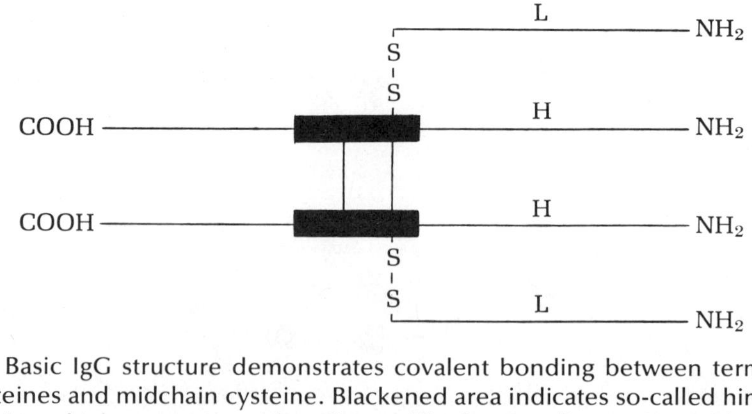

Fig. 1-17. Basic IgG structure demonstrates covalent bonding between terminal light chain cysteines and midchain cysteine. Blackened area indicates so-called hinge region that contains a high percentage of proline and hydroxyproline amino acids.

A change in ionic strength (the concentration of ions) can interfere with electrostatic bonds. A change in pH, as we have seen, can induce random coiling. A change in pH may effect ionization and in turn effect hydrogen bonding. All of these alterations of the medium can cause denaturation of the protein, producing loss of specific activity. Denaturation is generally considered to be the unfolding of polypeptide chains and can be caused by anything that would interfere with the formation of tertiary structure. A denatured protein will often renature or resume its native state when returned to its normal physiologic environment. The activity returns when the protein resumes its native conformation.

Have we come full circle? Are we again speaking of an unassembled watch rebuilding itself? This denatured, unfolded, untwisted protein can resume its native shape when returned to an appropriate environment. Again we look at the question—what is different about this protein that endows it with this self-constructing quality? Every piece of a watch has *one* unique characteristic shape. Each amino acid has a family of unique characteristics that make it respond in a particular way. Certain amino acids are hydrophobic while others are hydrophilic; some are large and others are small and unobtrusive, and some may be positively charged while others are negatively charged. Energy is provided to the unfolded and untwisted protein by the molecule's perpetual search for stability. This energy thrusts the unassembled protein into its natural conformation, which is indeed its most stable and active form.

PROTEIN ACTIVITY

Specific ligand binding is the most common functional characteristic of proteins. Recognition and specific binding of ligands have represented a fascinating challenge to scientists since the 1800's. Ehrlich first applied the now popular lock and key concept to the binding of antigen and antibody. He described antibody as a lock with a particular well-organized and specifically shaped binding region. The key, he felt, was the antigen with its complementary shape. The crux of this lock and key model was its complementary nature. The initial use of this concept is attributed to Emil Fisher in the 1890's. Fisher applied the complementarity of the lock and key geometry to the reaction of enzyme with substrate (Fig. 1-18). The simplistic lock and key model still holds some attractive features. Of major importance in this model is an emphasis on the "active site" region. On the surface of protein molecules, amino acids make up the "active site" region. These amino acids are responsible for binding and recognition of ligand. Both Fisher and Ehrlich hypothesized that a complementary geometry was responsible for specific ligand binding. Today we know that although structural geometry may be important in ligand binding, it is chemical complementarity that is ultimately most dominant. Complementary molecules interact not merely via geometry but rather charge, hydrophobicity, and hydrogen bond susceptibility. As shown in Fig. 1-19, recognition and specific ligand bonding occurs through the interaction of protein amino acids with the ligand molecule. Those

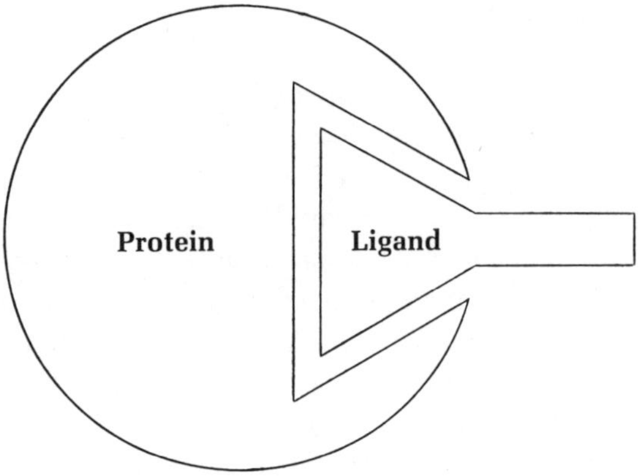

Fig. 1-18. Complementary geometry of the "lock and key" model for ligand binding by protein.

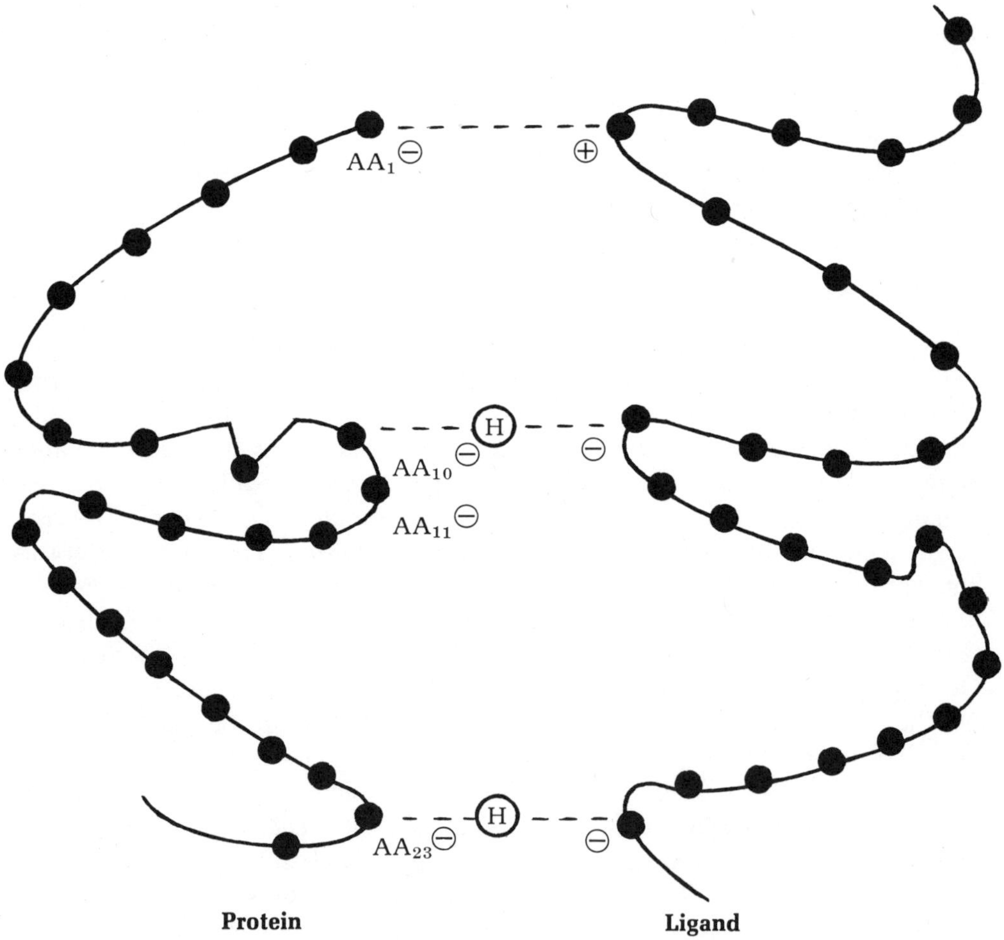

Fig. 1-19. Modern lock and key interpretation. Note amino acid sequence is critically important to binding.

forces that brought amino acids 1, 10, 11, and 23 to their juxtaposition are ultimately responsible not only for structure but activity.

METHODS FOR CHARACTERIZATION OF PROTEINS

The techniques used to isolate, quantitate, and characterize proteins are fundamental to any study of protein chemistry. Many of the procedures discussed are used in the preparation of reagents. The techniques of protein chemistry frequently are utilized in clinical assays.

Solubility

Protein remains in solution due to the interaction of hydrophilic R-groups with water. In a process known as salting out, various protein fractions may be precipitated. As one adds salts to protein solutions, the salts become preferentially hydrated. The continuous addition of salt yields progressive dehydration of proteins. The resultant decrease in available water to interact with proteins causes precipitation of protein. This process can be used to selectively precipitate protein fractions. For example, 28% sodium sulfite-sulfate will precipitate all globulins and leave only albumins in solution. Since proteins are not denatured in this process, rehydration will return protein to its native state. Repeated precipitation procedures are frequently used in the initial attempts to purify protein, and usually this step is followed by procedures with higher resolution. Salt fractionation techniques are sometimes used in the clinical laboratory to fraction serum proteins into albumins (A) and globulins (G). Total protein normally ranges 6 to 8 gm/dl (grams per deciliter) with the A/G approximately 1.8 to 2.0. As can be seen in Table 5, there is significant clinical value in assessing protein fractions. Generally stated, albumins are soluble in water and may be precipitated by saturated salt solution, while globulins are not soluble in water. Globulins are most frequently precipitated with a 50% saturated salt solution. Serum proteins are a heterologous group of proteins with at least a hundred fractions. Salt precipitation, at best, represents a crude assessment of any particular fraction. Clinical medicine and modern research demand more precise techniques of separation.

Table 5. Variation in serum albumin and globulin fractions in pathologic states*

	Nephrosis	Multiple myeloma	Infectious hepatitis	Cirrhosis	Systemic lupus erythematosus
Albumin	Low	Normal	Low	Low	Low
Globulin	High	High-normal	High	High	High
Total protein	Low	High	Low	Low	Normal

*Modified from data from White, W. G., Erickson, M. M., and Stevens, S. C.: Chemistry for the clinical laboratory, St. Louis, 1976, The C. V. Mosby Co.

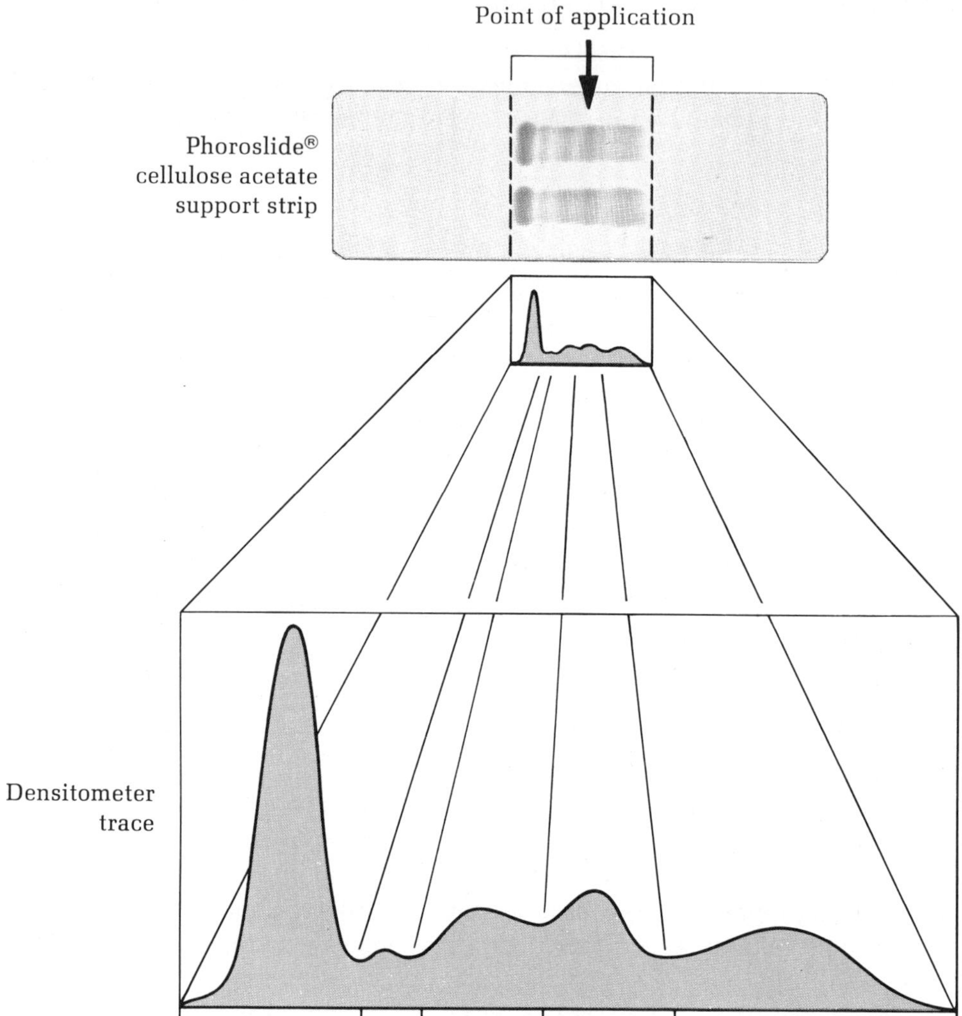

Fraction	Albumin	α_1	α_2	β	γ
% total concentration	52-68	2.4-5.3	6.6-13.5	8.5-14.5	10.7-21.0
gm/dl	3.6-5.0	0.1-0.4	0.5-1.0	0.6-1.2	0.6-1.6

Fig. 1-20. Illustration of protein electrophoretic separation of serum fractions. (Reprinted with permission of Millipore Corporation, Bedford, Massachusetts.)

Table 6. Visual comparison of serum electrophoretic fractions and functional characteristics

Electrophoretic fraction	Normal per-cent composition	Functional proteins
Albumin	60	Transport, osmolality
Alpha-1	5	Prothrombin, enzymes, protein
Alpha-2	8	Prothrombin, enzymes, protein
Beta	12	Lipid carriers, hormones, some antibody
Gamma	15	85% antibody and chylomicrons

Electrophoresis

During the past 20 years the necessity for greater resolution of protein fractions has led to a rapid expansion of electrophoretic techniques. In the most general terms, electrophoresis is the separation of charged particles in an electric field. Proteins are colloidal particles and at an alkaline pH of approximately 8 to 9 all serum proteins have a net negative charge. When placed in an electric field, these charged particles will move toward the positive electrode. The rate of movement of the particle will depend on several factors:

1. Size and shape of particles
2. Type of support media
3. Charge on particles
4. pH of the buffer
5. Temperature
6. Strength of force of the electric field
7. Ionic strength of the buffer

As shown in Fig. 1-20, a serum sample is placed on a cellulose acetate or agarose support medium and is buffered at a pH of 8.6. At this pH albumin becomes most electronegative and moves most rapidly in the charged field. The use of zone electrophoretic techniques has allowed a closer evaluation of protein fractions. As can be seen in Table 6, the clinician is able to assess many of the physiologic capabilities of proteins along with protein changes that may occur with certain pathologic conditions.

The use of polyacrylamide gel as a support medium increases resolving power sharply and allows accurate evaluation of 50 protein fractions (Fig. 1-21). Electrophoresis is a versatile technique and can be used on a variety of clinical and nonclinical specimens. Protein studies are frequently done on a myriad of bodily fluids including serum, urine, and spinal fluid.

Isoelectric focusing

Isoelectric focusing is a powerful analytic tool that isolates fractions and simultaneously determines the isoelectric point of each fraction. As previously dis-

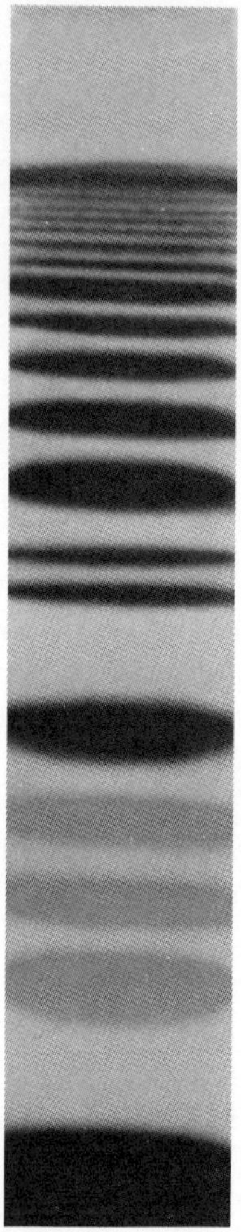

Fig. 1-21. Polyacrylamide electrophoretic fractionation. (Duplicated with permission of Ames Company, Elkhart, Indiana.)

cussed, molecules at the pH of their isoelectric point have a neutral charge and do not migrate in an electric field. The principle of this technique, as with many valuable techniques, is simple. The sample is merely electrophoresed through a pH gradient. As can be seen in Fig. 1-22, a protein buffered at pH 8.6 would move down the gradient until it reaches its pI. At the pI of each fraction the proteins assume a neutral charge hence migration stops. Isoelectric focusing is used to isolate and purify protein fractions. The fields of immunology and enzymology have made extensive use of this method to isolate relatively homogenous immunoglobulins or enzyme preparations.

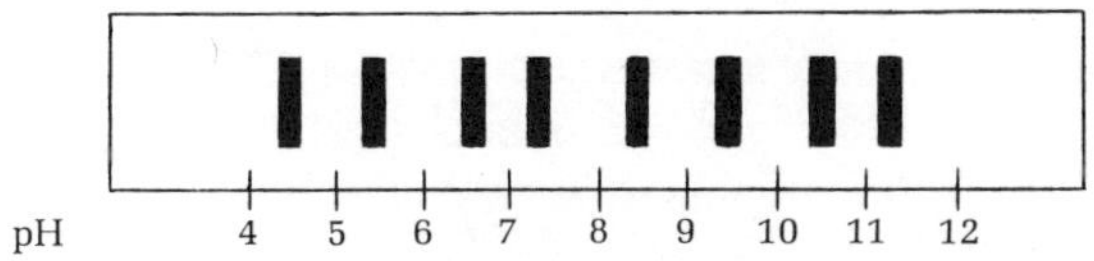

Fig. 1-22. Rough diagrammatic representation of isoelectric focusing. Protein is electrophoresed through pH gradient. Each protein fraction comes to rest at its particular isoelectric point, as indicated by blackened rectangles.

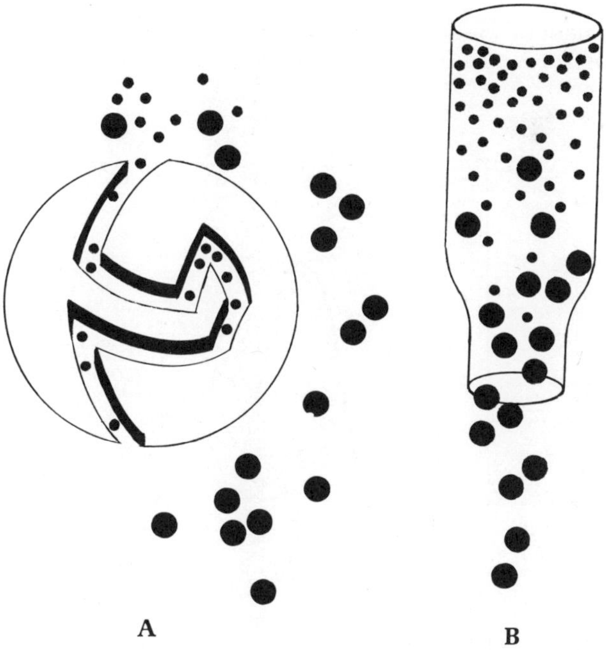

Fig. 1-23. Diagrammatic representation of gel bead fractionation. **A,** Hindrance of small particles as they pass through the beads. **B,** Gel column. Large molecules elute first.

Gel filtration

Molecular sieving is analogous to gel filtration. It is a process of separating molecules primarily by size. Gels, such as Sephadex (Pharmacia Biochemical Corporation, California), are high molecular weight cross-linked dextrans formed into beads. These beads are purchased with a specific pore size. A pore of an appropriate size will allow all molecules smaller than that pore into the bead. In entering the bead the molecule faces a slow arduous journey. Those molecules larger than the pore rapidly slip around the bead. These gels are frequently packed into glass columns. The gel columns are washed with buffers and carefully overlaid with sample. As can be seen in Fig. 1-23, the first fraction eluted from the column would contain the larger molecular weight molecules. A major

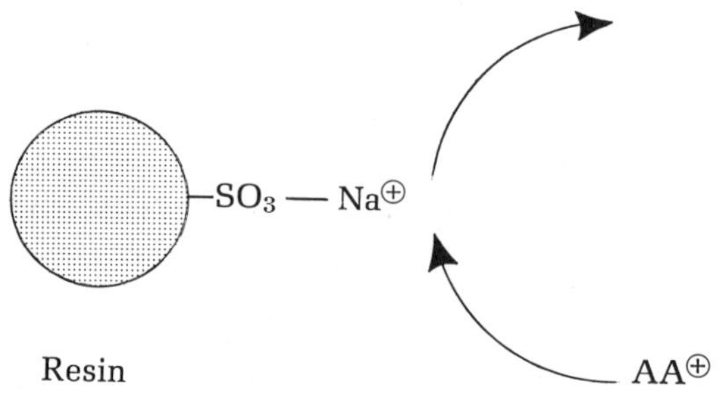

Fig. 1-24. Displacement of sodium ion, in ion exchange chromatography, by more positively charged substances. AA indicates amino acids.

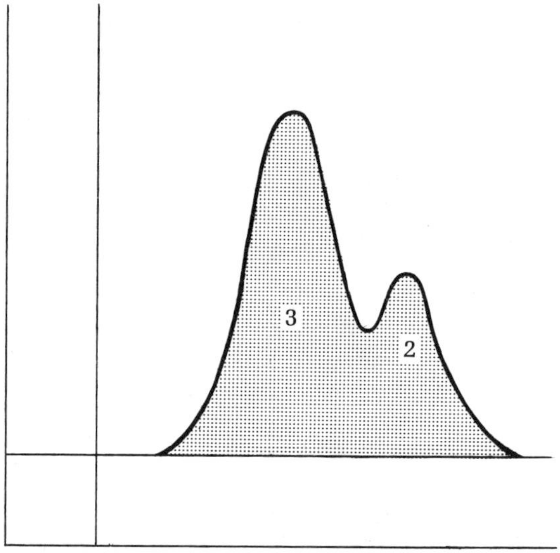

Fig. 1-25. Creatine phosphokinase (CPK) isoenzymes can be separated by ion exchange chromatography. CPK II, "MB" band, is specific for cardiac muscle. Percentage of CPK II increases during heart damage in a myocardial infarct.

advantage of gel filtration in separating proteins is that the mild environment of the column does not affect conformation or activity. It is possible with gel filtration to separate protein fractions and then test each for activity. Gel filtration is presently an invaluable tool to research and in the preparation of specific antisera or enzymes.

Ion exchange chromatography

Many substances are ion exchangers. These substances weakly bind a particular ion and will readily give it up in exchange for another type of ion. For example, polystyrene-sulfonated resin, equilibrated with NaOH, has sodium attached by weak electrostatic forces. A molecule with a greater positive charge will rapidly displace sodium and bind to the resin.

A protein at an acid pH would be positively charged and may displace sodium (Fig. 1-24). If the pH was raised slowly, according to the "protonic equilibria," the pH at some point would reach the pI of each protein. That protein would loose its charge and would then be released from the bead. These beads are also packed into columns. Ion exchange columns are used clinically to separate isoenzymes as shown in Fig. 1-25.

Ultracentrifugation

The ultracentrifuge is primarily a powerful research tool. Current interest in identifying a so-called floating lipid band in type III hyperlipidemia has given increased diagnostic value to this instrument. Macromolecules centrifuged at rapid speeds (such as 760,000 rpm) sediment or migrate at a rate dependent on the overall size and shape of molecules. The unit of measure used is S, the sedimentation constant. The S unit is a characteristic constant for a particular molecule under given conditions.

READINGS AND RESOURCES

Anfinsen, C.: Principles that govern the folding of protein chains, Science **181:**223, 1973.

Dickerson, R. E., and Geis, I.:The structure and action of proteins, New York, 1969, Harper & Row, Publishers.

Kendrew, J.: The three dimensional structure of protein molecules, Sci. Am. **205:**96, 1961.

Lehninger, A.: Biochemistry, molecular basis of cell structure and functions, ed. 2, New York, 1975, Worth Co.

Merrifield, R. B.: The automatic synthesis of proteins, Sci. Am. **218:**56, 1968.

Pauling, L., Corey, R. B., and Hayward, R.: The structure of protein molecules, Sci. Am. **191:** 51, 1954.

Stein, W. H., and Moore, S.: The chemical structure of proteins, Sci. Am. **204:**81, 1961.

Wold, F.: Macromolecules: structure and function, New Jersey, 1971, Prentice-Hall, Inc.

Zeffren, E., and Hall, P.: The study of enzyme mechanism, New York, 1973, John Wiley & Sons, Inc.

CHAPTER 2

Immunoglobulins

Immunoglobulins are a group of operational molecules synthesized by cells of the reticuloendothelial system. The stimuli for the synthesis of antibodies are biologic and chemical agents that the body recognizes as foreign. Antigens and antigenicity will be reviewed in Chapter 3. However, a basic definition of these terms is necessary to comprehend immunoglobulin synthesis and antibody specificity. An antigen has two major characteristics. It is capable of stimulating a specific immune response and of reacting with preformed antibodies. Some substances, usually of low molecular weight, are not capable of inducing antibody synthesis without the aid of carrier molecules. These incomplete antigens are called haptens and can react specifically with preformed antibody but cannot by themselves induce antibody formation. Like other operational molecules antibodies are capable of specific recognition and binding of ligand (antigen). The forces involved in this interaction are essentially the same as those of any operational molecule. Interaction of antigen and antibody may lead to the ultimate neutralization of the agent. This chapter will focus attention on: (1) antibody synthesis, (2) the research involved in the elaboration of the structure of IgG antibodies, (3) the classification of immunoglobulins, and (4) the antibody active site.

THEORIES OF ANTIBODY SYNTHESIS

Human serum protein content is approximately 6 to 8 gm/dl. Electrophoretic fractionation of serum proteins will separate essentially five major fractions: albumin, alpha$_1$, alpha$_2$, beta, and gamma. Although some antibodies are found in the alpha and beta globulin fractions, most antibodies are gamma globulins. There are two major theories of antibody synthesis, directive and selective.

Directive theory

The directive theory describes a response in which immunocompetent lymphocytes synthesize a protein, which folds on top of antigen. The antigen serves

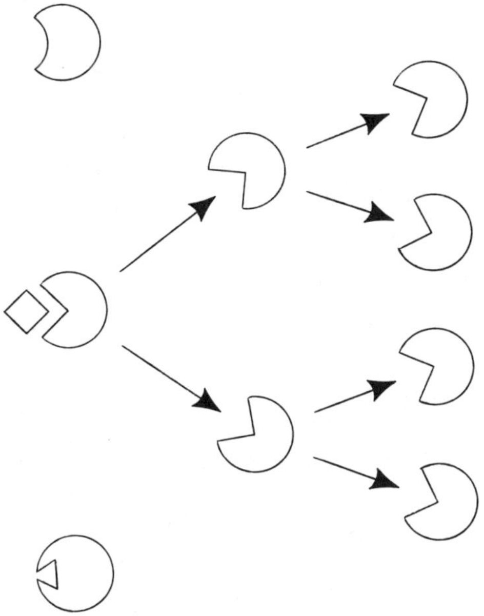

Fig. 2-1. Burnet's clonal selection model. Antigen binds to lymphocyte receptors with best "lock and key" fit. Binding stimulates antigen-sensitive cell to divide and differentiate into a clone of cells capable of responding to the initial antigen.

as a template dictating antibody shape or activity. Modern concepts of protein chemistry (that is, structure dictates function) are incompatible with this theory as stated. Recently, interest has grown in the directive theory owing to the discovery of mRNA-antigen complexes within lymphocytes. Although the idea of macrophage mRNA coupling with antigen to instruct lymphocytes in protein synthesis is exciting, it still appears to be contrary to the bulk of currently available evidence. The mRNA-antigen complex may act as an adjuvant to aid the immune response but it probably does not direct the response.

Selective theories

In the selective theories lymphocytes are committed to the synthesis of particular antibody. The specific antibody is on the surface of the lymphocyte and acts as a receptor for antigen. The binding of antigen to its complementary antibody-like receptor on the cell surface stimulates these cells to rapidly divide and differentiate. This stimulation produces a clone of cells that synthesizes antibody with a particular specificity (Fig. 2-1.)

Ehrlich is generally considered to be the father of selective theories, but Burnet is credited with the clonal selective model. There is a great deal of evidence to support and oppose both theories; however, our understanding of this complex problem is far from complete. What is known today is that this account is not nearly as simple as either the selective or directive models indicate. It is

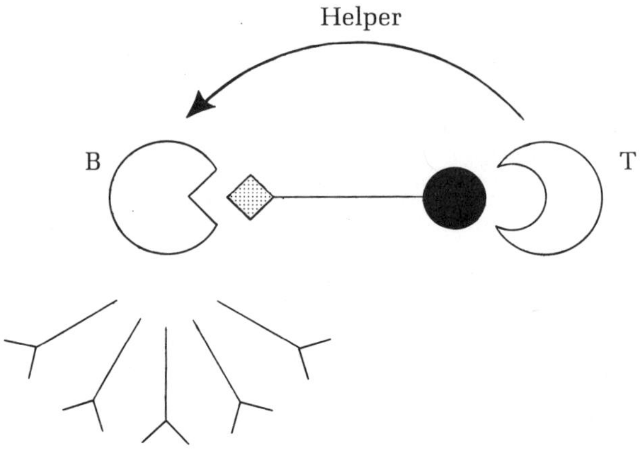

Fig. 2-2. T cell–dependent antigens bind to certain antigenic determinants while B cells react with other antigenic sites. The model demonstrates possible regulatory effect of T cell in enhancing antibody response to certain antigens.

now known that there are at least two major populations of antigen-sensitive lymphocytes, B cells and T cells with surface receptor sites. T cells are so termed because the stem cells from which they are derived pass through the thymus and are potentiated via thymic hormones, whence they emerge as thymus-dependent lymphocytes. B cells derive their characteristic behaviors via a precursor tour through an organ in birds called the bursa of Fabricius. In mammals the homologous lymphoid tissue responsible for B cell differentiation is thought to be the gut-associated lymphoid tissue (GALT). When either the B or T cells are eliminated, there is generally a loss of immunologic competence. The study of cell surfaces and receptors of such cells is in an explosive period of experimental development. It appears that T cells may bind certain determinants and release suppressor factors for self-antigens in order to suppress B cell autoantibody function. Helper factors exist to stimulate normal B cell antibody function (Fig. 2-2). As the complexity of antibody synthesis unfolds, it is clear that B cells primarily secrete antibody and that T cells appear to be regulatory. All the components of the lymphoreticular system must act cooperatively to provide the host with a normal immune response. The macrophage may play a role in concentration of antigen and direction of the immune response.

IMMUNOGLOBULIN STRUCTURE

Over 80% of the immunoglobulins belong to the IgG class. The Nobel Prize–winning work of Porter and Edelman elaborated the structure of this class of immunoglobulins. After enzymatic treatment with papain, Porter used ion exchange chromatography to characterize the digested immunoglobulin. As shown in Fig. 2-3, enzymatic treatment decreased the sedimentation coefficient from

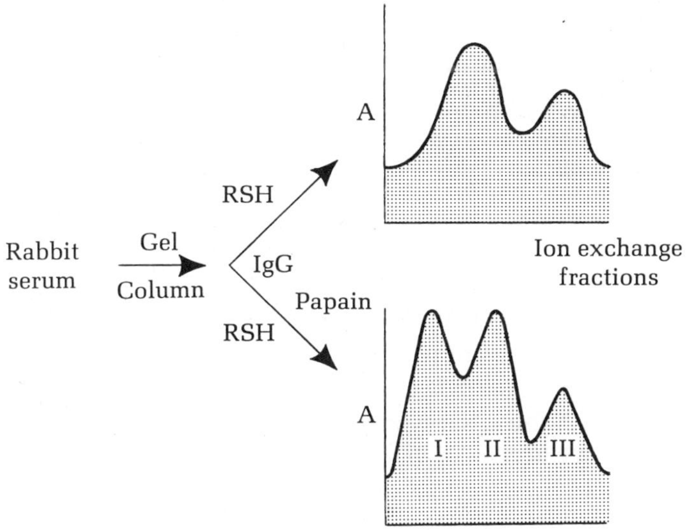

Fig. 2-3. Diagrammatic representation of Porter's Nobel Prize–winning research, digesting IgG antibodies to univalent fragments.

7.0S to 3.5S. When the absorption of ultraviolet light for the ion exchange fractions was plotted, a two-peak curve had been transformed into three peaks.

After enzymatic treatment, fragments I and II retain antigen-binding activity, hence the term "antigen-binding fragment (Fab)." The third fragment was similar in each study. It had no antigen-binding activity and was readily crystallizable, hence crystallizable fragment (Fc). Further studies showed that the Fab had a sedimentation constant of 3.5S and a molecular weight of 50,000 daltons.

In 1959, Edelman at Rockefeller University, New York, attempted to determine whether the antibody molecule is composed of a single chain by treating human IgG with mercaptoethanol, a mild reducing agent. After reduction the immunoglobulin had a sharp drop in molecular weight, suggesting a multiple-chain structure. After reduction the chains were exposed to 8 M urea to inhibit hydrogen bonding and refolding, and the protein chains were fractionated by electrophoresis. These studies indicated that IgG was composed of light (L) and heavy (H) chains. Since the molecular weight of the L chain was about 25,000 daltons, the H chain was about 50,000 daltons, and the total was 150,000 daltons, simple arithmetic led to the basic four-chain concept. The next question asked concerned the exact location of Porter's fragment in the four-chain structure. Antisera was prepared against rabbit IgG, Fab, and Fc and that antisera was tested with heavy and light chains. The reaction of H and L chains with antisera prepared against Fab and Fc fragments of rabbit IgG is shown in the boxed material at the top of p. 30.

	Antiserum to	
	Fab	Fc
H	+	+
L	+	−

As shown in Fig. 2-4, the model was complete; IgG is composed of two Fab regions and one Fc region. Antisera prepared against light chains did not react with all immunoglobulins. Immunizing animals with various L-chain preparations identified two types, lambda (λ) and kappa (κ). Each natural immunoglobulin contains only one or the other type but not both. It was later shown that the Fab and Fc regions tended to be compact and globular. However, the adjoining "Y" region is more linear, nonglobular, and is far more sensitive to enzymatic attack than the rest of the structure. More recent advances in immunoglobulin structure have been accomplished with rapid automated amino acid sequencing technique and x-ray crystallography. The greatest resource for the study of immunoglobulins is the unfortunate patient with multiple myeloma and related lymphoproliferative disorders. The serum from these individuals when subjected to electrophoresis shows abnormal fractions (Fig. 2-5).

Patients with multiple myeloma have monoclonal plasmacytic proliferation. This uncontrolled proliferation of a single clone of antibody-producing cells results in the patient having serum that has an extremely high concentration of antibody of a particular type and specificity. The specificity of these abnormal antibodies is rarely known. Myelomas have been found that elaborate all of the known classes of immunoglobulins as well as partial molecules, such as light chains. Immunoglobulin class IgM is produced excessively in a similar disorder, Waldenström's macroglobulinemia. These proliferative immunoglobulinopathies are associated with an increased serum protein containing monoclonal spikes. The urine of these individuals frequently has free light chains that demonstrate peculiar solubility patterns. These urine light chains will precipitate on heating and then, as the temperature rises, will redissolve. This urine protein is named after its discoverer, Dr. Bence Jones, and is known as Bence Jones protein.

CLASSIFICATION OF IMMUNOGLOBULINS—STRUCTURE AND FUNCTION

IgG

IgG antibodies are composed of two light and two heavy chains (Fig. 2-6). The heavy chains are antigenically specific for the class and are immunodominant. Injection of human IgG into a rabbit would result in antihuman-gamma antibodies that would be able to react with all human IgG. The amino acids are numbered from the amino terminal of light and heavy chains. During biosynthesis the amino end is synthesized first as occurs in the synthesis of all proteins. Completion of the amino acid sequencing of IgG led Edelman to propose his domain hy-

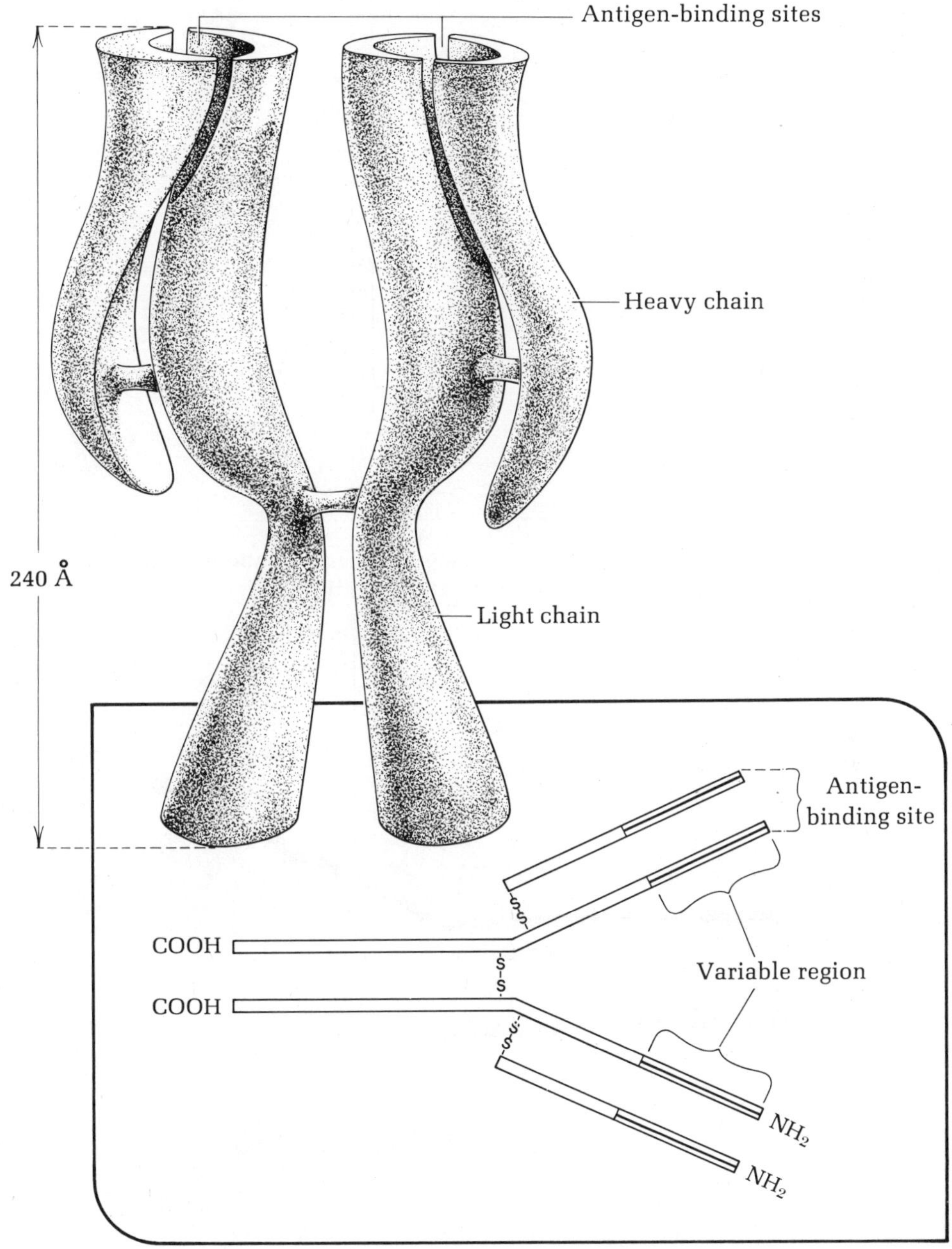

Fig. 2-4. Basic structure of antibodies of IgG class. (Reprinted with permission of Millipore Corporation, Bedford, Massachusetts.)

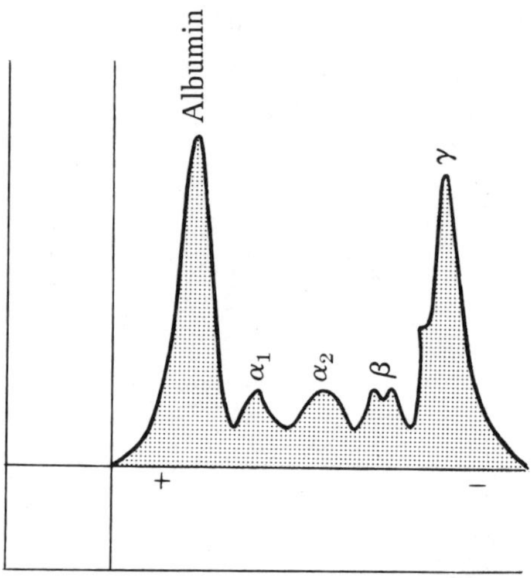

Fig. 2-5. Protein electrophoresis of serum specimen from patient with multiple myeloma. Note gamma region is excessively greater than normal.

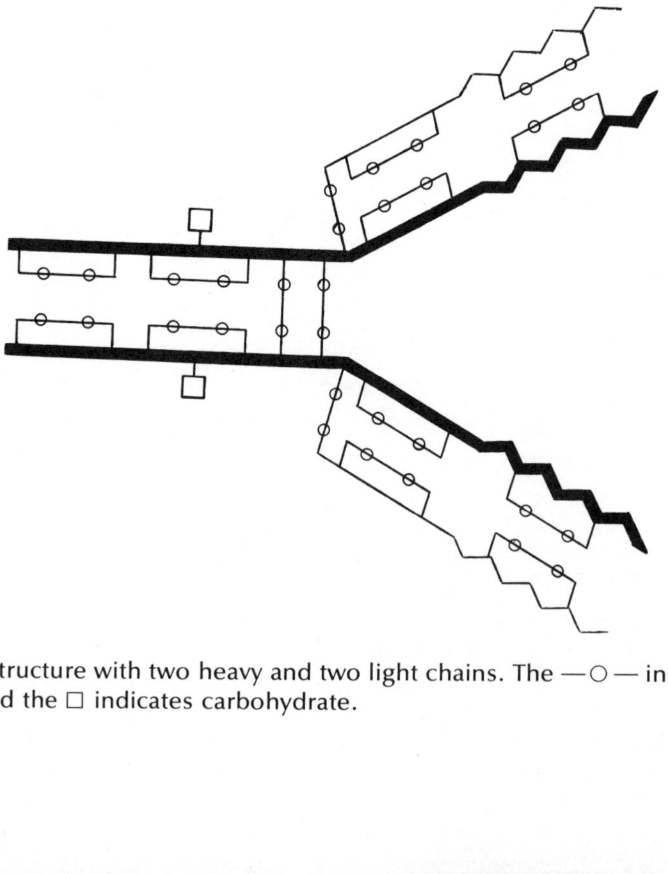

Fig. 2-6. IgG structure with two heavy and two light chains. The —○— indicates disulfide bonds and the □ indicates carbohydrate.

pothesis. Edelman noted repeating sequences of approximately 110 amino acids, which have a high degree of similarity or homology within a sequence. For example, within each 110 amino acids there exists one 60 AA loop formed via a highly resistant intrachain disulfide bond. The carboxyl end of the light chains and the carboxyl end of heavy chains all have an extremely high degree of homology, and the amino acid sequence was common to other mammalian immunoglobulins. The amino end of light and heavy chains has greater heterogeneity within certain areas, resulting in hypervariable regions. Each IgG molecule has two light chains and both are either kappa or lambda. The light chains have a carboxyl terminal cysteine, which covalently links to cysteines within the mid area of the heavy chains; this is the nonglobular hinge region, rich in proline and hydroxyproline. Several studies have shown at least three hypervariable regions within the light chains. Genetic variations in light chains produce amino acid changes at certain positions, creating genetic allotypes. Those genetic markers in the kappa chains are called Inv markers. Nonallelic markers in lambda chains are found in what is called the Oz region. Genetic variations in the heavy chains produce amino acid substitutions, which create genetic allotypes. These markers (Gm) are inherited by mendelian genetic ratios.

Heavy chains are composed of four, 110 amino acid domains. It appears likely that evolution, through gene duplication, added domains to perform specific functions. The first variable domain of the heavy chain bears a striking resemblance to the light variable region. It was believed that heavy chains were totally responsible for antigen binding. Today we know that maximum binding requires the combined effect of both light variable and heavy variable areas. There are three constant domains in the carboxyl end of heavy chains. Using proteolytic enzymes on IgG antibodies, Edelman found no loss of antigen binding but did observe changes in secondary immunoglobulin functions. Edelman proposed that each disulfide loop within the polypeptide chain of immunoglobulins forms globular domains with unique functional characteristics. Enzymatic cleavage of immunoglobulins causes a loss in affector functions. If C_H2 is removed, the serum protein complement cannot be bound or activated. Enzymatic cleavage of the C_H2—C_H3 junction with plasmin results in loss of macrophage adherence. Macrophages have receptor sites for the C_H3 portion of certain immunoglobulins. These act not only to aid in localizing and concentrating antigen for presentation to lymphocytes but they also aid in phagocytosis.

In the midregion of heavy chains (the so-called hinge region) between C_H1 and C_H2, there is a sequence of 15 amino acids. These 15 amino acids have been shown to contain a high percentage of prolines and hydroxyprolines. One of the most characteristic features of these two amino acids is that they are alpha helix breakers. Proline and hydroxyproline keep this region of the molecule somewhat linear, allowing limited rotation. Bending within this heavy chain region gives it a hingelike function. The term "hinge region" is frequently used to identify that particular area responsible for bending. The lack of globular conformation and coiling in this region increases the accessibility to the hinge from outside molecules. The proteolytic enzymatic digestion carried out in Porter's studies occurred because of the linearity of the hinge. The bending of the hinge has been observed by electron microscopy.

The exact structural formula for IgG is $\gamma_2\lambda_2$ or $\gamma_2\kappa_2$. IgG is synthesized at a rate of 20 to 40 mg/kg/day; its biologic half-life is approximately 27 days, and it normally reaches a serum level of 800 to 1600 mg/dl. In the normal adult about 50% of the IgG is concentrated in the extravascular space. IgG is capable of crossing the placenta. Radioactive-tagged IgG experiments have shown, however, that transport across the placenta must be active and unidirectional, mother to fetus. Each IgG molecule has two active sites giving a theoretical valence of two. In vitro studies have proven IgG capable of binding two antigenic sites. Occasionally, an immunologist or immunohematologist may refer to a univalent IgG antibody. There are several reasons why an IgG may appear univalent. Univalency is more likely to represent monogamous binding than true univalency; that is, the two active site regions on a single antibody bind to different sites on the same antigen molecule.

The IgG molecule is considered remarkably stable due primarily to the high number of hydrogen bonds and disulfide covalent bonds. After unusually large changes in temperature, pH, and ionic strength, this immunoglobulin, if returned to its normal environment, will regain native conformation and original activity. IgG antibodies are resistant to reduction with mercaptoethanol unless first denatured with urea. Studies on IgG human myeloma proteins have demonstrated four antigenically distinct subclasses of the gamma chain. The four IgG subclasses, as shown in Table 7, have functional variations. Considerable homology is seen in all IgG subclasses with characteristic determinants in the Fc region.

IgA

IgA antibodies are polymeric molecules and can exist as monomers, dimers, an even trimers, of the basic four-chain structure. The monomer is 7S, the dimer is 9S (Fig. 2-7), and the trimer is 11S. The IgA molecule is capable of cross-linking antigens. Under the conditions of mild reduction, as with mercaptoethanol, this cross-linking capability is lost. This mercaptoethanol treatment study indi-

Table 7. Comparison of functional variation in IgG subclasses

	IgG1	IgG2	IgG3	IgG4
Complement fixation	+	+	+	−
Alternate complement pathway	−	−	−	+
Macrophage adherence	+	±	+	±
Capable of placental transfer	+	±	+	+

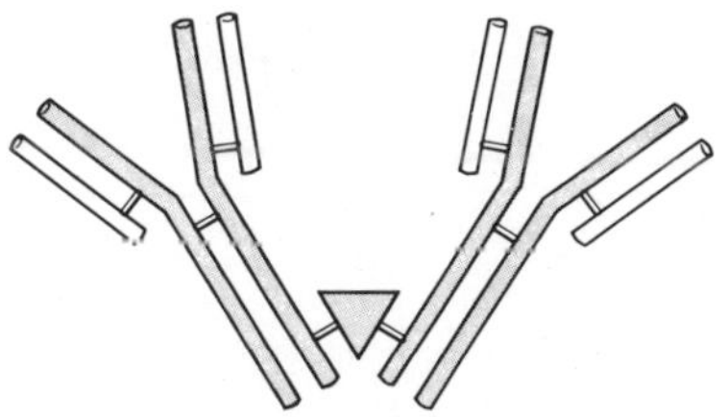

Secretory IgA

Fig. 2-7. Basic structure of secretory IgA. (Reprinted with permission of Millipore Corporation, Bedford, Massachusetts.)

cates the presence of disulfide bonds. The basic IgA monomer is structurally similar to IgG. IgA does not bind complement and therefore is incapable of activating complement via the classical pathway. This class of immunoglobulins possesses approximately 10% carbohydrate, and the dimer has a molecular weight of about 320,000 daltons. The half-life of IgA is 7 days, and the rate of synthesis is approximately equal to that of IgG, 2.4 gm/day. With this rapid rate of synthesis the average serum value of 225 mg/dl is far below what would be expected. The low serum value is primarily due to the rapid catabolic pace of IgA degradation. IgA, like some other immunoglobulins, has extra structures not present on IgG. Evolution has provided immunoglobulins with these structures to tie monomers together and to aid in secretion and transport across membranes. The multimeric IgA has a so-called joining piece or J piece. One J piece exists per four light chains. Exocrine IgA is the primary immunoglobulin on all mucous surfaces in exocrine secretions. Exocrine secretions contain high concentrations of enzymes, many proteolytic, which would destroy most immunoglobulins. Secretory IgA is equipped with a 60,000 dalton molecular weight multiple polypeptide, which many speculate may function to protect the sensitive immunoglobulin hinge. The ambiguity existing around the purpose of this structure is best seen by the names given it, such as secretory piece and transport piece. Those that call this structure a transport piece believe it responsible for the secretion of IgA molecules across mucous membranes. Several genetic variants of the heavy alpha chain exist and are responsible for the AM allotypes of IgA. IgA antibody is capable of binding complement via classical pathway and appears responsible for the defense of bodily "ports of entry."

IgM

While IgG antibody is best known for its ability to precipitate antigen, IgM can best agglutinate or lyse the antigen. The normal adult, with a rate of IgM synthesis of 3 to 17 mg/kg/dl, reaches an IgM blood level of 50 to 200 mg/dl of serum. IgM molecule consists of five, 7S, four-chain, IgG-like subunits. These subunits are linked by disulfide bonds and J chains. The normal IgM pentamer

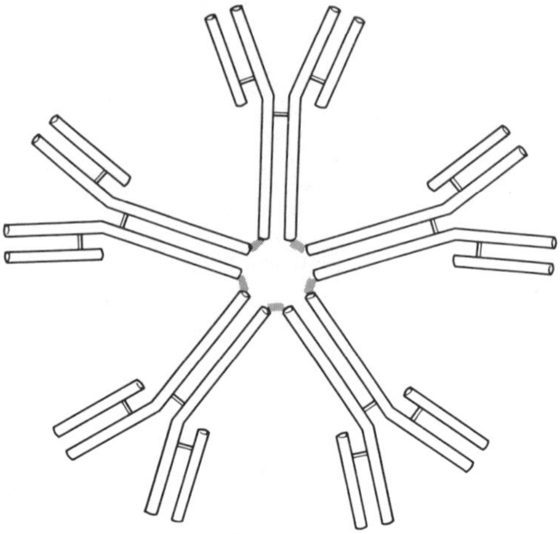

Fig. 2-8. Basic structure of IgM. (Reprinted with permission of Millipore Corporation, Bedford, Massachusetts.)

structure is 19S, but 23S and 7S conformations do exist. IgM antibodies have an electrophoretic mobility between beta and gamma globulins. This macroglobulin is incapable of placental transfer, but its multimeric structure makes IgM an excellent activator of complement. The antigenically distinct, heavy μ chain is larger than the heavy chains of IgG and IgA antibodies. The μ chain has five domains and a molecular weight of 70,000 daltons. IgM antibodies are frequently synthesized in response to nonprotein bacterial antigens in the early immune response. The theoretical valency of 10 gives IgM antibody an advantage in the battle against infection. The intact IgM molecule (Fig. 2-8), however, is capable of binding at five sites. This valence discrepancy is thought to be due to the steric hindrance within the giant IgM molecule. The agglutinating power of IgM, which requires cross-linking of antigens, is lost with mild mercaptoethanol treatment. A monomer of IgM is similar to IgG. Since IgG antibodies are also capable of cross-linking antigen, researchers were faced with a new dilemma. The two Fab fragments of an IgM monomer have unequal binding strength with the antigen site, which must play a role in determining the binding power of IgM. The avidity, the strength of binding, per Fab fragment within an IgM monomer is low and unequal. The molecule as a whole demonstrates a "bonus" effect. Simply stated the bonus effect indicates that the binding of several Fab fragments to separate antigenic sites on a single molecule sharply raises the avidity. Massive increases of IgM are most frequently encountered in the serum of patients with Waldenström's macroglobulinemia. Occasional increases in IgM are noted in patients with certain lymphoproliferative and infectious disorders.

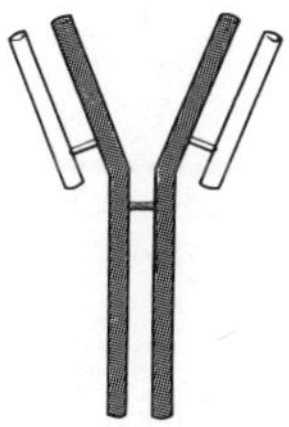

IgD

Fig. 2-9. Basic IgD structure. (Reprinted with permission of Millipore Corporation, Bedford, Massachusetts.)

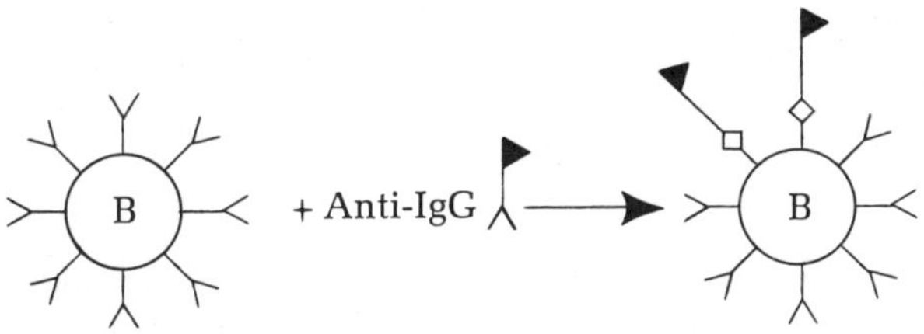

Fig. 2-10. Reaction of fluorescent anti-IgG with IgG-coated B cells. Flag (▶) indicates areas that fluoresce under ultraviolet light and can be seen by fluorescent microscopy.

IgD

IgD immunoglobulins were discovered in a patient with an unusual myeloma protein. This class of immunoglobulins was found to constitute an extremely small fraction of the total serum immunoglobulin in the normal individual. The adult total serum IgD concentration is equal to approximately 3 mg/dl and it is synthesized at a rate of 0.03 to 1.5 mg/kg/day. IgD antibodies are structurally similar to other immunoglobulins with either kappa or lambda light chains and its own antigenically distinct heavy delta (δ) chains. The delta chain has a molecular weight of 77,000 daltons. As shown in Fig. 2-9, IgD like IgG has two Fab fragments. IgD antibodies are composed of approximately 15% carbohydrate and have a sedimentation constant of 6.8S. The exact role of IgD in immunity has been elusive and most certainly the present state of knowledge concerning its role is incomplete. Researchers using extremely sensitive and mild radioassay techniques have proposed that IgD is a major immunoglobulin on the surface of lymphocytes. Many studies on cell surface immunoglobulins have identified molecules of IgG, IgA, IgM, and IgE, but not IgD. These latter studies all used antibodies directed to immunoglobulins with fluorescent tags. The fluorescent-tagged antiantibody allowed visualization of surface immunoglobulin when viewed under a fluorescent microscope. As shown in Fig. 2-10, visualization of the fluorescent tag indicates the presence of the specific antibody on the lymphocyte surface. According to Vitetta and Uhr, IgD may be the infamous antigen

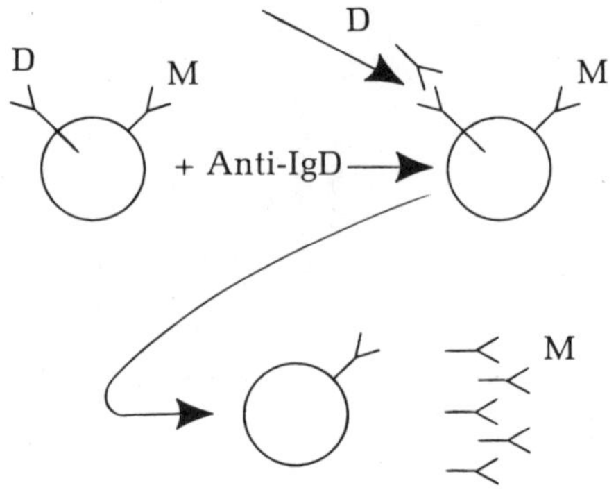

Fig. 2-11. Hypothetical pathway, illustrating surface IgD buried within lymphocyte surface along with surface IgM. Reaction of antigen or antiantibody with IgD results in enzymatic cleavage of IgD and degradation in circulation. B cell then is transformed into active antibody-synthesizing plasma cell.

receptor trigger. They propose, convincingly, that when IgD binds immunologically to antigen, a conformational change is induced in IgD molecule. The conformational change of surface IgD exposes the Fc region to enzymatic attack. Cleavage of IgD stimulates antibody production (Fig. 2-11). Since others have failed to find surface IgD, Vitetta and Uhr incorporated this ambiguity in their model. Another theory holds that there is only one disulfide bond between the heavy chains of IgD, and the instability of this bond prevents isolation of the intact molecule. At present, it has not been determined whether elevations of IgD are pathologic or are related to any particular disorder. Some researchers have suggested a correlation of IgD to rheumatoid arthritis and systemic lupus erythematosus. IgD antibody is found normally in cord blood of the newborn.

IgE

In 1967, Johansson and Bennich characterized an 8S immunoglobulin that did not cross-react with antisera prepared against purified IgD, IgG, IgM, and IgA. Ishizaka and others found that the 8S immunoglobulin was the long-sought, skin-sensitizing reagin found in patients with asthma and other allergic conditions. IgE antibody has a molecular weight of 200,000 daltons and demonstrates the basic four-chain structure of IgG. The epsilon (E) heavy chain has a molecular weight of 75,000 daltons and has an extra Fc domain. As other immunoglobulins, IgE has either two κ or two λ light chains. IgE is 8.2S; it has approximately 11% carbohydrate with a valence of 2. In the normal individual IgE is synthesized at a rate of 0.2 mg/kg/day. This synthetic rate, coupled with a short circulating half-life, accounts for the normal low serum concentration of 10 to 90 ng/dl. The short circulating half-life is due to the high affinity of the Fc of IgE to receptors on mast cells or basophils (Fig. 2-12). IgE is synthesized by mature lymphocytes (plasma cells). Upon release from plasma cells, IgE quickly binds

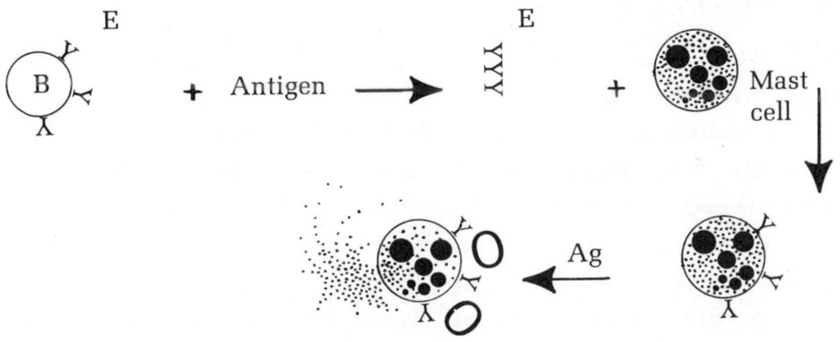

Fig. 2-12. Probable pathway for release of potent pharmacologic mediators. Plasma cells on antigenic stimulation may synthesize antibodies of IgE class. IgE antibodies fix to receptors on mast cells, platelets, and basophiles. Binding of antigen on second exposure to antigen results in release of mediators.

Table 8. Comparison of structure and function of immunoglobulins

	IgG	IgA	IgM	IgD	IgE
Mol wt × 1000	150	150-300	900	180	200
Sedimentation coefficient	7S	7S-11S	19S	6.1S	8.2S
Half-life (days)	25	8	8	6	8
Carbohydrate content (%)	2.5	10	10	–	10
Valence	2	2	5-10	2	2
Subclasses	4	2	–	–	–
Placental transfer	+	–	–	–	–
Complement activation	++	–	++++	–	–
Adult normal concentration (mg/dl)	1200	225	125	3	90 ng/dl
Mercaptoethanol resistance	High	Moderate	Low	High	–

its Fc region to basophil or mast cell receptors. The extended Fab fragments remain capable of binding antigen with the original specificity. Binding of antigen to cell-bound IgE can serve to cross-link the surface IgE and appears to trigger the release of potent pharmacologic mediators (Fig. 2-12). These mediators bring about the signs and symptoms of hypersensitivity, such as smooth muscle contraction, hypersecretion, and increased vascular permeability. Although the total serum IgE is always a mere fraction of the total immunoglobulin level, there is no doubt that it is a major immunoglobulin responsible for allergic hypersensitivity. As will be discussed in later chapters, quantitation of serum IgE and determining its specificity are of great value to the allergic patient and represent a major challenge to the clinical laboratory. A comparison of immunoglobulin classes is shown in Table 8.

IMMUNOGLOBULIN SYNTHESIS

Autoradiography is a sensitive technique that enables researchers to visualize protein synthesis. This technique utilizes radioactive amino acids. Antibody-synthesizing cells are cultured with the radioactive amino acid–enriched media. The tagged amino acids are incorporated into the newly synthesized polypeptides. Layering these cells with photographic emulsions allows visualization of protein synthesis. Energy released from the isotopic decay is sufficient to expose the photographic emulsion and when developed provides an image of protein synthesis. Using autoradiography it was shown that light and heavy chains were synthesized on separate polysomes and that the variable and constant regions were produced in one linear sequence. The light chains, with their approximately 214 amino acids, complete synthesis faster than do heavy chains. Synthesis begins at the amino end. The last amino acid of the light chains, the carboxyl terminal amino acid, is cysteine. The light chain cysteine covalently links with the cysteine in the incomplete heavy chain. An enzyme, glucosyl transferase, adds carbohydrate to the heavy chains that are still incomplete. A particular amino acid sequence acts as the substrate to direct carbohydrate addition. The light-heavy pair covalently bonds to a separate light-heavy pair, resulting in a complete four-chain immunoglobulin monomer. The finished immunoglobulin drains into the Golgi apparatus via the endoplasmic reticulum. In the Golgi apparatus the antibody is stored prior to secretion. The exact mechanism for the secretion of antibody is not totally clear. Secretion is antigen driven and most probably is related to microtubular function and the cAMP/cGMP ratio. Impairment of secretion may constitute one of an array of immunodeficiency diseases that will be discussed later.

ANTIBODY-COMBINING SITE

The antigen-binding site, the active site in antibody, is that part of the antibody that interacts with antigen. As other types of ligand binding, such binding is not a process of antibody binding to antigen but rather antibody interacting with antigen. The active site is approximately 1% of the total surface area of the immunoglobulin molecule. In studies employing x-ray crystallography it has become possible to carefully examine the fine structure of immunoglobulins, measure exact distances between atoms, and observe the conformation. The major drawback, besides cost and complexity, is that it is dependent on crystallization of the molecule under study. Using a polyglucose-binding myeloma protein and x-ray crystallography, the active site was found equivalent to the size of approximately six glucose molecules or 20 Å (the equivalent of 10 to 20 amino acids). Does antibody specificity and binding depend on amino acid sequence? To determine the answer, IgG was denatured with 8 M urea. The unfolded molecule was then reduced with mild mercaptoethanol to disrupt disulfide bonds. Upon reduction, the antibody lost most, if not all, antigen-binding activity. As with earlier studies on protein renaturation, antibody resumed its native conformation and binding specificity when the cysteines were allowed to reform covalent bonds through oxidation. This experiment, done with a heterologous antisera (an antiserum with a mixture of antibody specificities), can be used to produce a bivalent antibody.

It was thought that antibody binding was primarily due to heavy chain activity. After preparing antibodies to simple haptens the antibody was purified, denatured, and reduced. The mixture was then passed through a gel column to separate light and heavy chains. Once separated the light and heavy chains were immobilized on beads and put into a glass column. The hapten suspension was then passed through light chain columns and heavy chain columns and hapten retention was determined. The objective of the study was to determine if light chains could bind hapten, and if they did, would that binding be stronger or weaker than heavy chain binding. Light chains did bind hapten although the retention was not as great as with heavy chains. The study showed that light and heavy chains are involved in hapten binding.

A technique known as affinity labeling is used in an effort to identify the precise amino acids involved that interact with hapten or antigen. In this technique a reactive hapten is used with a specific antibody. The reactive hapten is unstable, and when it is bound to antibody, strong covalent bonds result instead of the usual weak interactions. If the antibody is then hydrolyzed, the resultant amino acid pool would contain certain amino acids with covalently bound hapten. With enzymatic digestion and amino acid mapping techniques it becomes possible to identify the amino acids involved in binding and their location. Recently, researchers studying antibody specificity have begun to question some of the long-established basic concepts of immunology. Many of these studies have tested antibodies in experiments that paralleled work done on enzyme specificity. It is now realized that although enzymes are somewhat specific their specificity is far less than once believed. The importance and implications of these studies require us to review the data in some detail.

How specific is antibody? Is the specificity of antibody absolute? Any person studying immunology or using antibodies in analytical procedures must, at some time, address antibody specificity. Researchers in the field of immunology, both biochemical and clinical, have established major tenets concerning antibody activity. Many of these basic rules were developed by Landsteiner over 30 years ago.

1. Antibodies are specific for the antigens that elicit them.
2. Antibodies may or may not cross-react with structurally related antigens.

These two ideas alone have profound implications. For example, to the immunogeneticists and molecular biologists it means that any theory of antibody production must contain in it a mechanism for the production of one antibody for every different antigen. A clone of cells must result in order to produce an antibody to every antigen. We must account for where all the DNA might come from and why evolution would have provided animals with clones of lymphocytes and DNA dedicated to antibody synthesis directed at artificial haptens.

As frequently happens, a simple observation led to the radical changes of today's theories of antibody specificity. It was shown that tadpoles, with only 10^6 lymphocytes, are capable of building a specific detectable immune response to dinitrophenol (DNP). The importance of this observation may be missed unless you are aware of two adjacent rules.

1. One clone is necessary to produce one type of antibody.
2. In the tadpole 10^5 lymphocytes are needed to build a detectable response.

Simple calculations and reasoning tell us that if all the above are correct then our tadpole could only respond to ten antigens. It seems ridiculous that tadpoles may respond with a detectable antibody response to only ten antigens. This paradox is compounded by the fact that one of the ten responses was shown to be for a synthetic hapten, dinitrophenol (DNP). The inference is that tadpoles' lymphocytes are multipotential or, alternately, antibody must be capable of binding with multiple specificities.

Recently hapten binding by myeloma proteins has become a valuable tool for the study of binding specificity. Using these homogeneous immunoglobulins, it is possible to show that antibody is capable of distinguishing differences of only a single atom in the structure of the hapten. At the same time it can be shown that these immunoglobulins can bind totally unrelated diverse molecules.

To emphasize the diverse binding characteristics of immunoglobulins, researchers tested a mouse IgA myeloma protein. They found this immunoglobulin capable of a high degree of discrimination. It bound DNP well but did not react with trinitrophenol (TNP) or mononitrophenol (MNP) as shown in Table 9. Although the mouse immunoglobulin could easily distinguish a single NO_3 group, it bound strongly to a totally unrelated molecule, menadione (MD).

This study showed that a single immunoglobulin is capable of binding totally unrelated haptens but did not question where in the Fab region this may have occurred. It was unlikely that MD and DNP had similar complementary areas. Was it possible that DNP and MD bound at two distinct areas within the Fab region? Kabat in earlier efforts to measure Fab-reactive areas showed that binding took place in an area of 20 to 30Å, but could it occur at two separate sites? To test this problem researchers used chemical modifiers. These are substances that react with specific amino acids within Fab regions and inhibit binding of haptens. The inhibition is the key to the study. When the hapten no longer binds to immunoglobulin, the critical amino acids have been modified. When this

Table 9. Comparative binding activity of mouse IgA myeloma

	DNP	MNP	TNP	MD
Mouse IgA Myeloma	+++	–	–	+++

A

B

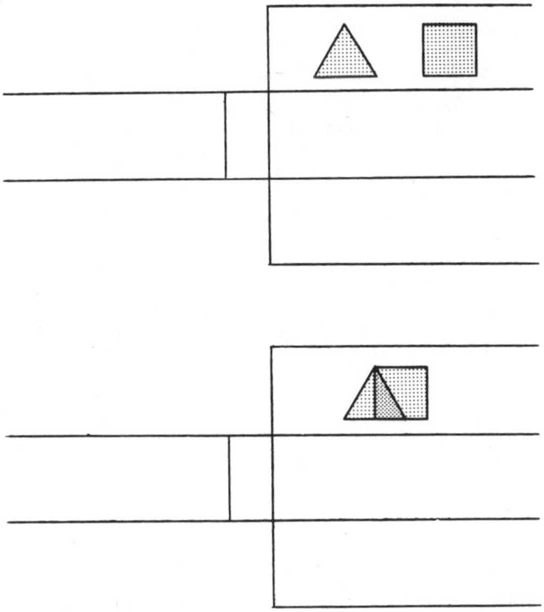

Fig. 2-13. Possible binding areas of DNP and MD to mouse IgA myeloma protein. **A,** Sites are separate and distinct. **B,** Sites for hapten binding overlap.

technique was used on mouse IgA, it was possible to inhibit binding of DNP but not MD. This chemical modifier inhibition study suggested that two or more sites may exist within a single antibody.

As can be seen in Fig. 2-13, *B*, the possibility still exists that altering a critically located amino acid may affect the binding of DNP but may not be so important to the binding of MD. This alternate suggestion keeps the overlapping binding area theory viable. The answer can be found only by measuring exact dimensions of binding areas. The complexity and problems in crystallization led researchers to a second method, fluorescent energy transfer, to determine these dimensions.

As light travels a certain distance there is a precise loss of energy; this principle is utilized in fluorescent energy transfer (Fig. 2-14). A fluorescent molecular probe is attached to a reference point. This probe is chosen for its unique fluorescent characteristics. The first probe used must be able to emit light of a particular wavelength when it is exposed to ultraviolet light. The emitting wavelength must be that wavelength needed to induce fluorescence in MD. In a similar manner a second probe that will be capable of exciting DNP is chosen, and it is attached to the reference point. With the use of a complex trigonometric formula and a means to determine the energy emitted by bound DNP and MD, it is possible to calculate binding dimensions. This fluorescent study proved that MD and DNP bind at distinct sites at least 14 Å apart and that binding regions on

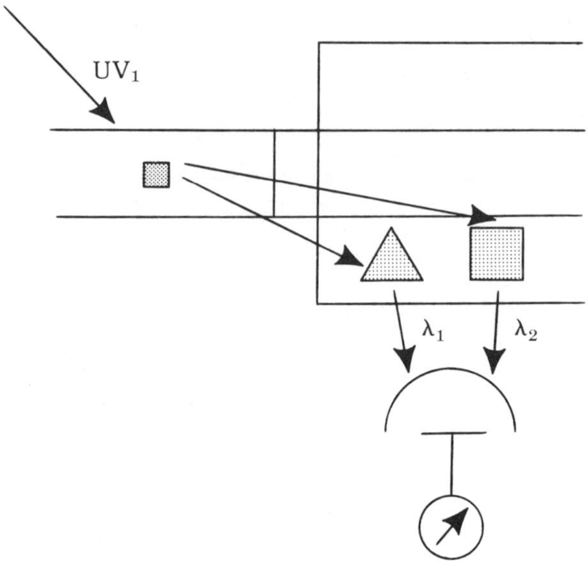

Fig. 2-14. Diagrammatic representation of the use of fluorescent probes to calculate areas of hapten binding. Energy traverses the polypeptide causing hapten excitation-emission.

mouse IgA were not overlapping. To better comprehend the significance of this study one must remember that DNP and MD are two haptens that were found reactive with mouse IgA. It is possible that the same homogeneous myeloma protein may bind hundreds of totally unrelated ligands.

Recent efforts to crystallize mouse and human Fab myeloma proteins have been successful. This success has made it possible to perform x-ray crystallographic study of hapten binding. These crystallographs show that the cleft between light and heavy chains can be modulated by hapten binding. The modulation would result in exposing hidden amino acids of the antibody to ligand. This concept of antigen-induced modulation of antibody parallels Koshland's "induced fit" concept in enzyme-substrate reactions.

These experiments on specificity all show a multispecificity of myeloma immunoglobulins, but does this all represent artifact? The crucial question remains is antibody polyfunctional in vivo? Realizing that specific binding of antigen to B cell surface immunoglobulin is at least one of the triggering steps of antibody synthesis, Richards, at Yale, set out to test the polyfunction theory. Rabbits that had been shown to produce anomalous cross-reactions with particular haptens were used in his experiments. The rabbits were immunized with hapten-A protein complex. The response elicited was a spectrum of anti-A antibodies from numerous clones of lymphocytes. Each anti-A antibody had slight differences in activity and specificity (Fig. 2-15). Two portions of such antisera obtained from a single rabbit were subjected to isoelectric focusing. Each isolated

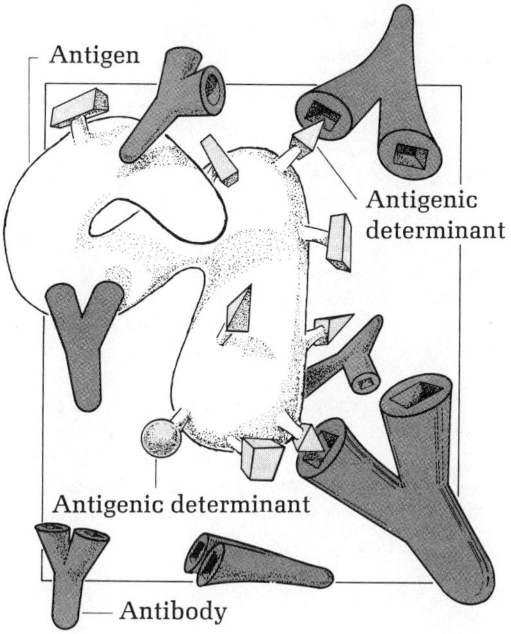

Fig. 2-15. Heterogeneity of antibody response to simple antigens. Note multiclonal response. (Reprinted with permission of Millipore Corporation, Bedford, Massachusetts.)

band from one of these duplicate samples was tested to identify all anti-A antibodies. The locations of these anti-A bands were determined by reactions with an antigen and used to remove anti-A from the remaining duplicate. The anti-A bands from the second isoelectric focusing preparation were then tested with the supposed anomalous cross-reacting hapten-B. The word "anomalous" is used because the rabbit was not immunized with hapten-B, yet it appeared to develop a specific response to B. A few bands were found that reacted with both hapten-A and hapten-B but the reaction was always stronger with A. If this antibody was capable of binding A and B, then maybe it was polyfunctional. Richards then immunized this same rabbit with hapten-B and closely monitored the antibody response. The rabbits always responded on initial B immunization with an increase in those isoelectric focusing bands that responded to A and B. Further, the early response of anti-A and anti-B was always stronger for hapten-A than for the immunizing hapten-B. These studies imply that the cell surface receptor, like the secreted immunoglobulin, is polyfunctional and capable of binding unrelated ligands. Assuming that all of the data and their implications are correct, immunologists must scrutinize the basic concepts long held as fact.

1. Antibody is specific for eliciting molecule.
2. When cross-reactions occur, the reaction is strongest with the eliciting molecule.

3. Cross-reactions occur because of
   a. Contaminating antigens
   b. Structurally related sites on the antigen
   c. Common determinant groups on the antigen

RESOURCES AND READINGS

Edelman, G. M.: The structure and function of antibodies, Sci. Am. **223:**34, 1970.

Edelman, G. M., and Gally, J. A.: Model for 7S antibody molecule, Proc. Natl. Acad. Sci. USA. **51:**846, 1964.

Eisen, H.: Immunology, New York, 1974, Harper & Row, Publishers.

Fahey, J. L.: Antibodies and immunoglobulins; structure and function, J.A.M.A. **194:**183, 1965.

Ishizaka, K., and Ishizaka, T.: Immunoglobulin E, current status and clinical laboratory applications, Clin. Chem. **100:**289, 1976.

Landsteiner, K.: The specificity of serological reactions, rev. ed., New York, 1962, Dover Publications, Inc.

Marx, J.: Suppressor T cells: role in the immune regulation, Science **18:**245, 1975.

Raff, M. C.: Cell-surface immunology, Sci. Am. **234:**30, 1976.

Richards, F. R., Konigsberg, W. H., Rosenstein, R. W., and Varga, J. M.: On the specificity of antibodies, Science **187:**130, 1975.

Vitetta, E. S., and Uhr, J. W.: Immunoglobulin—receptors revisited, Science **189:**964, 1975.

CHAPTER 3

Antigens and antigenicity

Circular definitions are often used to define antibody. "An antigen is any substance which stimulates the production of antibody." "An antibody is a protein synthesized upon antigenic stimulation." These definitions provide us with little insight into the nature of either antigens or antibodies. Searching the literature one finds another frequently used definition of antigen ". . . an antigen is a foreign protein which when parenterally administered to man, causes the production of antibodies." This latter definition, although much improved, is misleading. In this chapter the nature of antigens and antigenicity will be investigated for the purpose of building a new, more valid definition of antigen. Several terms will be introduced and clarified including immunogen, hapten, immunogenicity, and antigenicity.

NATURE OF ANTIGENS

Chemical composition

Empirically, proteins were found to be excellent antigens, but today immunologists realize that many substances can be antigenic. Man produces antibody to the exocellular polysaccharides of many bacteria. The antibodies that are induced act as clues in the identification of infection. Pneumococcal organisms are also capable of stimulating an immune response. Specific antisera prepared via pneumococcal immunizations have given man the capability of classifying the pneumococcus organisms into 88 serotypes. The complex lipopolysaccharide of *Salmonella* and *Shigella* organisms is an excellent example of nonprotein-antigen effectiveness in humans. After infection with these gram-negative bacteria, specific antibody may appear in collected serum samples. "A" and "B" substances, which are responsible for man's major blood group antigens, are all glycoproteins. Nucleic acids frequently act as antigens in both normal people and in patients with autoimmune disorders, resulting in antibodies to nucleoprotein, DNA, and RNA. It should be obvious that while antigens can be protein they are not always protein.

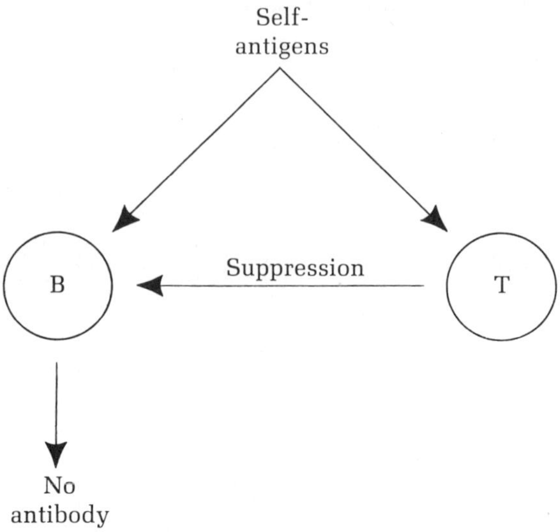

Fig. 3-1. Hypothetical model demonstrating interaction of B and T cells to suppress autoantibody response.

Phylogenetic foreignness

Immunologists experimenting with immunization techniques found that animals produced the best antisera when the antigen was from a phylogenetically distant animal. More importantly, they noted no antibody production to self-antigens (autoantibodies). The host animal is able to distinguish self from nonself through the complex interaction of the regulatory T cells and B cells. As seen in Fig. 3-1, self-antigens are identified by both lines of cells. B cells prepare to transform into antibody synthesizing plasma cells, while T cells distinguish antigen as foreign or self. If antigen is foreign, a helper factor may stimulate antibody production. If the antigen is recognized as nonself, a suppressor factor may inhibit antibody production as proposed by the Herzenbergs. The use of the term "foreign" in the definition of antigen requires modification. Many examples can be shown in which self-antigens are recognized as foreign and result in the production of autoantibodies. This situation arises in many states that cannot be considered pathologic, as in the elderly or after vasectomy. Table 10 lists several situations where autoantibody formation is frequently encountered.

When autoantibody synthesis does occur, it usually is the result of one of three reasons: (1) The animal or individual may have an intrinsic defect in the immune system that hinders its ability to distinguish self- and foreign (nonself) antigens, for example, a T cell deficiency. (2) Self-antigen can be modified by infection, injury, or drugs. After modification these self-antigens are different and can be recognized as foreign. (3) Certain self-antigens are normally sequestered from the immune system. Antigens, such as those from the cornea, if exposed to the circulatory system by injury, are then recognized as foreign and stimulate an

Table 10. Comparison of autoantibodies and their homologous self-antigens found in a variety of states

Antigens	Antibody	Disorder
DNA	Anti-DNA	Systemic lupus erythematosis
IgG	IgM-anti-IgG	Rheumatoid arthritis
Heart	Anti-heart muscle	Myocardial infarction
Thyroglobulin	Anti-thyroglobulin	Thyroiditis
Sperm	Anti-sperm	Vasectomy, infertility

immune response. Certain patients with hyperthyroidism have "hot nodules," hyperactive growths in their thyroid glands. These patients are candidates for surgery. During surgery the sequestered thyroid colloid, known as thyroglobulin, is released into the blood and may stimulate an immune response. Once sensitized, the immune system may continue to attack the now normal thyroid, leading to destruction of normal thyroid tissue resulting in hypothyroidism.

Animal host

The inclusion of "man" into the classical definition of antigen, that is, "a substance when injected into man, causes . . . ," suggests that a substance is only an antigen when it stimulates an antibody response in man. The earthworm has been shown to reject transplants. Antibodies of the IgM class have been detected in all vertebrates, down to the lowest living vertebrates, the jawless cyclostomes, hagfish, and lamprey and slime eels.

Mode of administration

Antigen need not be parenterally administerd. Polio vaccine is given orally to provide maximum protection to the gastrointestinal tract, the site where the polio virus normally sets up a primary infection. Allergic responses show some of the best nonparenteral modes of immunization: food allergies via the gastrointestinal tract, conjunctivitis due to dust and particles in the air, asthma via inhalation of allergens, and dermatitis merely through skin contact with allergens. Many of these nonparenteral routes of immunization bring about detectable levels of circulating antibody. Particulate substances tend to make better antigens than soluble substances, as can be seen when attempts to raise antibody to bovine serum albumin fail. However, heat denaturation of albumin may enhance antigenicity.

Function of antigen

Antigens have two major functions, and any definition of antigen must include both functions. An antigen is able to generate an immune response and react with the products of that response, cellular and humoral.

ANTIGENICITY AND IMMUNOGENICITY

Immunologists are now using two terms to describe antigen function. Immunogenicity is the ability to generate an immune response, and antigenicity is the capacity of the substance to react with antibody. Both terms are relative and many factors affect both functions. A complete antigen is an immunogen and an antigen; that is, it stimulates an immune response and reacts with antibody and lymphocytes, the primary cells of the immune system. An incomplete antigen or half-antigen (hapten) is a substance that is unable, by itself, to stimulate an immune response but is able to react with preformed antibody. When an incomplete antigen is attached to a helper or carrier molecule, the new complex behaves as a complete antigen. The antibodies formed as a result of immunization with this hapten carrier will be directed at various sites on the complex. Some of the antibodies will be specific for the low molecular weight hapten. The unconjugated hapten is capable of reacting with preformed antibody.

Definition of antigen

Antigens generally have a molecular weight of at least 10,000 daltons. The degree of immunogenicity usually increases with molecular weight. The shape or conformation of antigen is at least as important as the shape of antibody. Specific binding and recognition is dependent on the orientation of atoms within both antigen and antibody. Molecular complexity, stability, and structural rigidity vary directly with immunogenicity. A highly complex low molecular weight molecule will be more immunogenic than a giant homopolymer. If a substance is digestible or can be solubilized, it will be a better immunogen. A particulate substance that is nondigestible is fated to be a poor antigen. A soluble antigen, however, can have its immunogenicity increased by attachment to a particle. Generally speaking, proteins, polysaccharides, and lipid exhibit decreasing antigenicity in the above order.

We have now dismembered the classical definition of antigen and looked at both what an antigen is and is not. We are now ready for a new definition. Usually, complete antigen is a macromolecule with internal and external structural complexity, which is recognized as foreign and is digestible. A complete antigen is capable of stimulating an immune response (immunogenicity) and of reacting with the products of the immune response (antigenicity), antibody, B cells, and T cells.

Antigenic determinants

The specific areas or sites on the antigen that elicit antibody response and antibody binding are called antigenic determinants. The elements that are most distally projected tend to be immunodominant and result in good binding. The number of antigenic determinants per antigen molecule is equal to the antigenic valence. Cryptic or hidden determinants exist that often are not exposed until after antigen digestion. Monovalent antigen is capable of reacting with antibody but is not capable of forming a lattice structure by binding with many antibodies.

Immunogenicity

The previous description of antigen treats immunogenicity as though it were a physical property of the antigen. Immunogenicity is a complex phenomenon. Many factors influence the degree of immunogenicity.

1. The physical properties of the antigen
2. The biologic system
3. The route of administration
4. The method of immunization

The physical properties of the antigen and how they affect immunogenicity and antigenicity have been discussed. A number of studies have shown that certain animals are good responders to a particular antigen, while other animals are not. The good response can be bred via mendelian genetics, and good response has been shown to be controlled by a set of genes appropriately called the immune response (IR) genes. In the poor responding animals, the antibody response to a particular antigen is independent of the antigen. The antigen may be protein, large, complex, and foreign yet produce no immune response.

Adjuvants

The route of antigen administration has a limited effect on immunogenicity. Feeding the antigen usually results in antigen destruction. Intravenous, intramuscular, or intraperitoneal injection usually results in complete distribution of antigen throughout the lymphatics. High concentrations and low concentrations of antigens frequently produce tolerance or immune unresponsiveness. Hence any route tending to produce a high blood level may be tolerogenic. The use of adjuvants provides the safest, most economical, and reliable method to immunize animals for the purpose of developing a high-potency antibody. Adjuvants are substances that assist or improve the response to an antigen. A wide variety of substances behave as adjuvants. Substances such as calcium phosphate, inorganic gels, and aluminum hydroxide all assist the animal in responding to antigen. The most widely used adjuvant in animals other than man is a water-oil emulsion developed by Freund. The use of mycobacteria added to Freund's adjuvant markedly increases the potency of weakly immunogenic substances. Adjuvant is not antigenic itself, yet it enhances the total immune response. It is thought that adjuvant functions by protecting antigen from destruction, allowing a low-level persistent immunization. Adjuvants induce inflammation, which in turn attracts a greater number of lymphoid and phagocytic cells to the area.

It should be remembered that antigen is as important as the antibodies in immunology. For many years serology, the study of serum components, dominated clinical immunology. The clinical immunology laboratory focused its attention on detecting antibodies against a suspected agent in the serum of the patient with infectious disease. Today, serology is giving way to clinical immunodiagnostics, a new and exciting world. The immunodiagnostics laboratory is able to test for an enormous selection of antigens and antibodies with picogram sensitivity. The exquisite sensitivity and specificity of these new assay systems is in part due to man's ability to trick animals into building an immune response to substances that are normally considered nonimmunogenic.

SELECTED READINGS AND RESOURCES

Barrett, J. T.: Textbook of immunology, ed. 3, St. Louis, 1978, The C. V. Mosby Co.

Eisen, H. N.: Immunology, New York, 1974, Harper & Row, Publishers.

Haurowitz, F.: Immunochemistry and the biosynthesis of antibodies, New York, 1968, John Wiley & Sons, Inc.

Kabat, E. A.: The nature of an antigenic determinant, J. Immunol. **97:**1, 1966.

Kabat, E. A.: Structural concepts in immunology and immunochemistry, New York, 1968, Holt, Reinhart & Winston.

Karush, F.: Immunologic specificity and molecular structure, Adv. Immunol. **2:**1, 1962.

Landsteiner, K.: The specificity of serologic reactions, Bacteriol. Rev. **31:**157, 1967.

Nezlin, R. S.: Biochemistry of antibodies, New York, 1970, Plenum Press.

CHAPTER 4

The interaction of antigen and antibody

The union of antigen and antibody is fundamental to most immunoassays. The split-second time period required for union of antigen and antibody will be magnified in an attempt to identify the variables that affect this critical moment. This chapter will aid in developing an appreciation of quality control in immunoassay procedures and should provide insight into the mechanisms of error. The principle of lattice formation will be used to describe the second phase of the immunologic reaction, aggregation. New terms introduced in Chapter 4 include, specificity, cross-reactivity, titer, zonal phenomena, prozone, postzone, lattice, union, aggregation, affinity, and avidity.

ANTIGEN-ANTIBODY REACTION

Is the antigen-antibody reaction like any organic chemical reaction? We think of specificity as being unique to immunologic reactions. Organic reactions do exert some specificity, and, as seen in Chapter 2, antibody demonstrates a spectrum of specificities to a variety of haptens and antigens. The antigen-antibody reaction frequently is manifested via the precipitation of insoluble complexes. In a similar reaction certain chemicals can result in precipitation but with some crucial differences. A more in-depth study of these reactions will provide a means to evaluate this difference. Equation 4-1 expresses a reaction between sodium chloride and silver nitrate and the ensuing precipitation of silver chloride.

$$NaCl + AgNO_3 \rightarrow NaNO_3 + AgCl\downarrow \qquad \textbf{(Eq. 4-1)}$$

Conveniently, this precipitation reaction resembles that of many antigen-antibody reactions. Fig. 4-1 diagrammatically shows the experimental design of a study that examines the relationship of concentration of reactants to the concentration of precipitate. In tube 4 (Fig. 4-1) all of the sodium chloride and silver nitrate react and are consumed in the formation of precipitate. There exists a one-to-one stoichiometric relationship in tube 4—2 ml of 0.4 M silver nitrate and 2 ml of 0.4 M NaCl. In the later tubes the concentration of sodium chloride is reac-

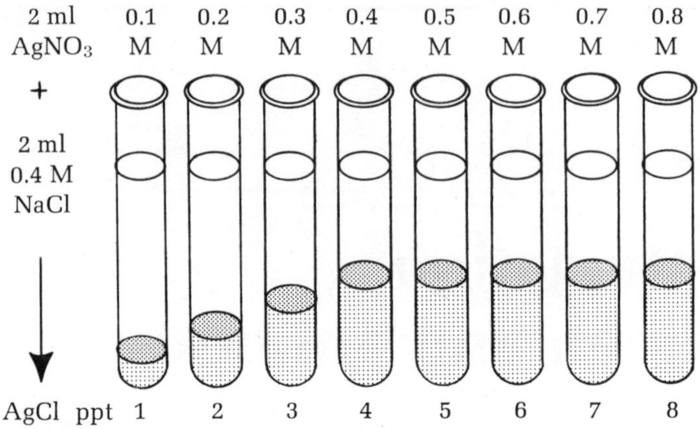

Fig. 4-1. Protocol of chemical precipitin reaction. In this experiment 2 ml of 0.4 M NaCl solution is added to eight test tubes. To each tube equal amounts of increasing con-concentrations of $AgNO_3$ are added, which results in formation of AgCl precipitation. Note dotted areas represent precipitate that increases in amount up to tube No. 4.

Supernatant from tube number

	(1)	(2)	(3)	(4)	(5)	(6)	(7)	(8)
NaCl	+	+	+	−	−	−	−	−
$AgNO_3$	−	−	−	−	+	+	+	+

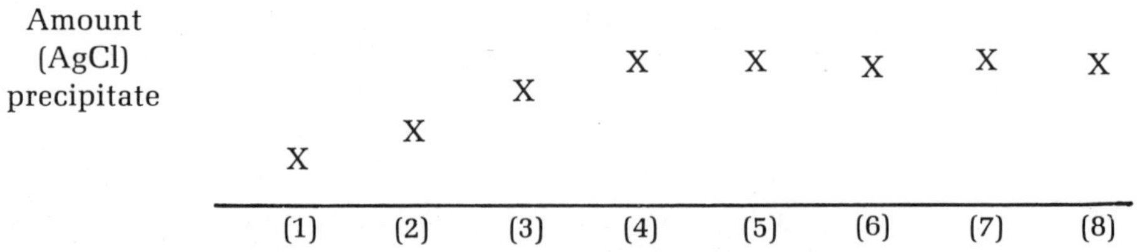

Fig. 4-2. Graphic representation of experimental data derived in Fig. 4-1. Note complete consumption of available NaCl in tube No. 4 with excess $AgNO_3$ present in tube Nos. 5 to 8. Maximum precipitation occurs in tube No. 4 and that level of precipitation is reached in tube Nos. 5 to 8.

tion limiting. There is no more sodium to react with the excess silver nitrate available. Careful analysis of the amount of precipitate formed in each tube and the presence of reactants in the supernatant lead us to some observations. (Note Fig. 4-2.)

Equation 4-2 shows the reaction of pneumococcal polysaccharide (pps) with a specific antibody (anti-pps). This reaction leads to the precipitation of insoluble complexes.

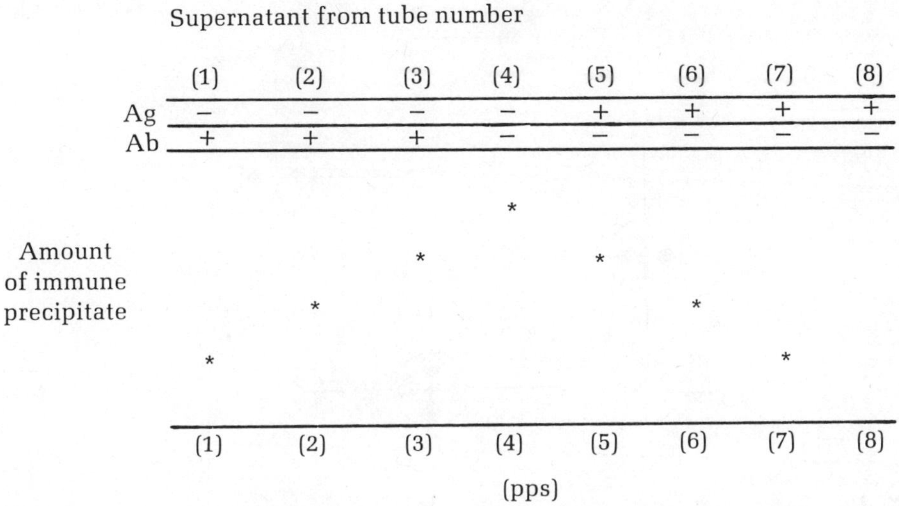

Fig. 4-3. Increasing concentrations of pneumococcal polysaccharide (pps) are added to eight tubes that contain equal amounts of specific antisera. Note that inhibition of precipitation is biphasic, tube Nos. 1 to 3 and tube Nos. 5 to 8.

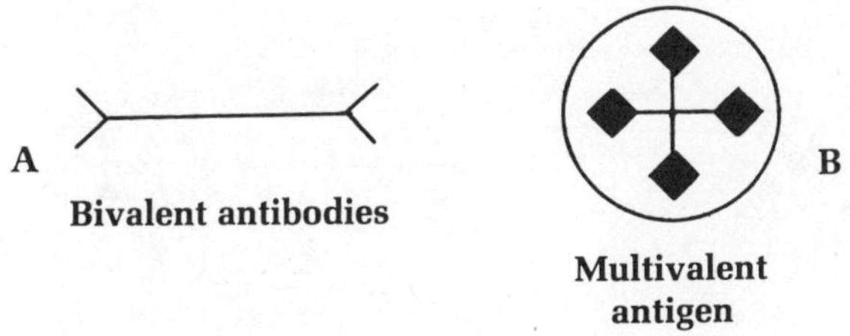

Fig. 4-4. Schematic diagrams depict valency of antigen and antibody. **A,** Bivalent antibody. **B,** Multivalent antigen.

$$\text{pps} + \text{anti-pps} \rightleftarrows \text{pps-anti-pps} \qquad \textbf{(Eq. 4-2)}$$

A protocol similar to that used in Fig. 4-1 was used to elaborate the data shown in Fig. 4-3. In comparing Figs. 4-2 and 4-3 some striking differences are noted. The most obvious and important difference is the dissociation of the complex formed in tubes 5 through 8. It appears that initially the reaction favors complex formation as is seen in equation 4-3.

$$\text{Ag} + \text{Ab} \rightarrow \text{AgAb} \qquad \textbf{(Eq. 4-3)}$$

Under increasing antigen concentrations, the reverse can occur as in equation 4-4.

$$\text{AgAb} \rightarrow \text{Ag} + \text{Ab} \qquad \textbf{(Eq. 4-4)}$$

If it were as simple as this, then we could explain this phenomenon merely

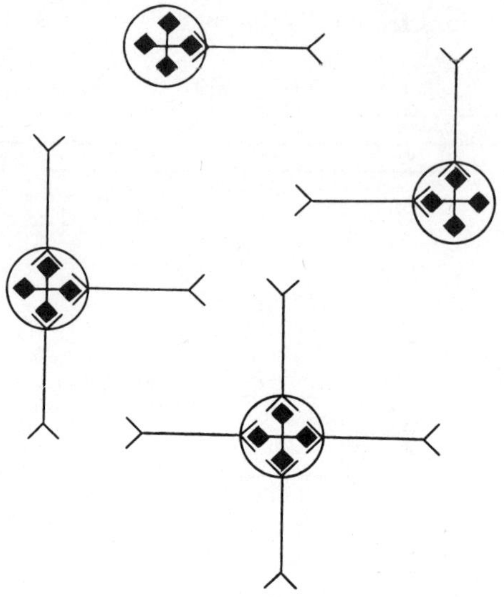

Fig. 4-5. Variety of binding ratios between bivalent antibody and tetravalent antigen.

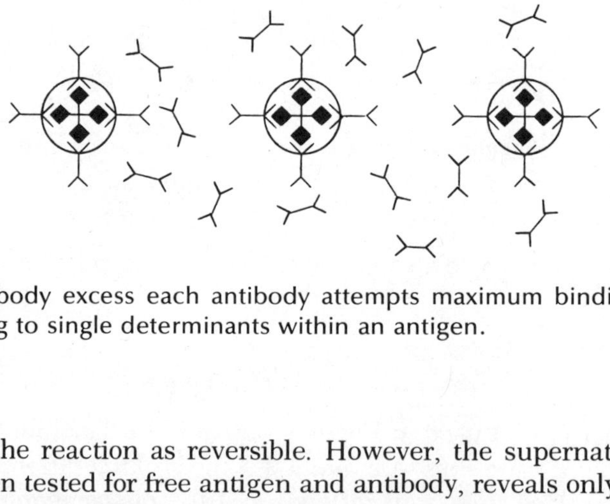

Fig. 4-6. In antibody excess each antibody attempts maximum binding, resulting in antibody binding to single determinants within an antigen.

by describing the reaction as reversible. However, the supernatant in tubes 5 through 8, when tested for free antigen and antibody, reveals only free antibody. The best explanation of this enigma comes in Marrack's lattice hypothesis.

Marrack, realizing that most antibodies are bivalent (IgG) while most antigens are multivalent, described a novel synopsis. Marrack reasoned that while most chemical reactions occurred at fixed reactant ratios, the antigen-antibody reaction was not limited to this requirement; for example, one molecule of bovine albumin may bind five antibody molecules. The multivalency of antigen and bivalency of most antibody favored variation in molar reaction ratios. Fig. 4-5 demonstrates this variation of antigen-antibody ratio, which becomes possible with a multivalent antigen and bivalent antibody. In the first few tubes of the

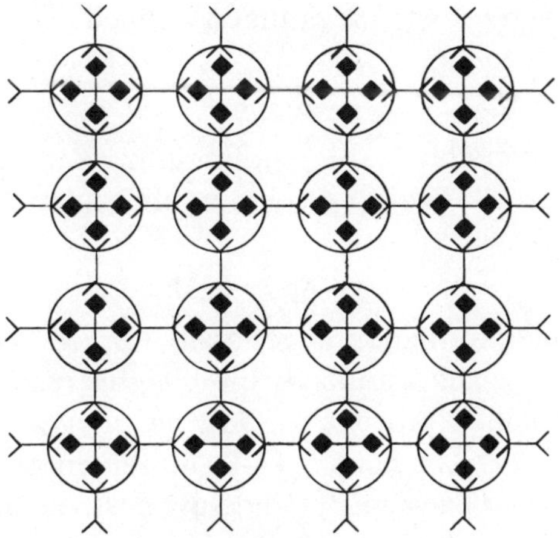

Fig. 4-7. At equivalence the ratio of antibody to antigen is such that all available reactants may be consumed in formation of lattice structure.

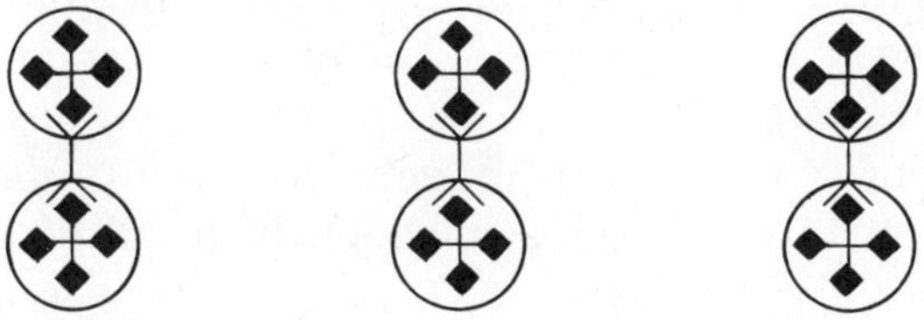

Fig. 4-8. Inhibition of lattice formation and precipitation occurs because of excess antigen.

immune precipitation study, there exists excess antibody. Since there is insufficient antigen, it is likely that each antibody will bind a single antigen. As the concentration of antigen increases, the ratio of reactants tends to shift. Each antibody molecule may bind two antigen molecules resulting in the development of an insoluble complex via lattice formation. At a high-antigen concentration one antibody may bind two antigens. Excessive amounts of antigen inhibit lattice formation as described in Fig. 4-8.

If an immune precipitate was isolated and more antigen was then added to the isolate, what would occur? At first, there would be no change, but shortly after the precipitate would go into solution. By adding more antigen the equilibrium is shifted and a situation occurs that favors solubilization of the complex. Precipitation of an immune complex, that is, four antibodies and one antigen or of a huge lattice complex is due to the exclusion of water from these complexes. If an immune complex has a decreased affinity for water due to the interaction of hydrophilic groups, then precipitation will occur. How can this be reversed? Our first observation with the study using pneumococcal polysaccharides and their specific antibodies was correct; the antigen-antibody reaction is reversible as shown in equations 4-3 to 4-5.

$$AgAb_4 + Ag \rightarrow AgAb_2^{(sol)} + AgAb_2^{(sol)} \quad \textbf{(Eq. 4-5)}$$

Since the reaction is reversible and in equilibrium, as in equation 4-6, the addition of antigen to the precipitate can lead to solubilization due to change in reactant ratios.

$$Ag + Ab \rightleftarrows AgAb \quad \textbf{(Eq. 4-6)}$$

Inhibition of complex formation is generally termed "zonal phenomena." In the early part of Fig. 4-3, excess antibody inhibits this reaction, hence the region of antibody excess is called prozone, indicating prior to the point of reactant equivalence. In the latter tubes of Fig. 4-3, inhibition occurs owing to excess antigen and is referred to as postzone, indicating postreactant equivalence. Aside from the specificity of the antigen-antibody reaction, we now find it is reversible and that the reaction is not limited to fixed molar reactant ratios.

Most reactions between antigen and antibody occur in two stages—the first of which is union. Union, the combination of antigen with antibody, has been shown to be one of the fastest reactions known to occur. Combination of antigen with antibody, as seen earlier, is due to interatomic, noncovalent interactions. Since a great number of antigens are protein, binding of these antigens may be, in effect, the partition of this protein antigen between an aqueous and nonaqueous phase. Nonspecific factors such as hydrophobicity of the antigen can greatly increase the rate of the forward reaction. The second stage of the reaction usually involves the visualization of the first stage, such as precipitation or agglutination. Lattice formation is a second-stage reaction that follows union. While union occurs in split seconds, the second stage may require minutes to hours or even days. The following is a list of basic suppositions of antigen-antibody reactions.

1. The reaction of antigen and antibody is specific.
2. The reaction of antigen and antibody is noncatalytically promoted.
3. Interatomic interactions occur between the active sites on antigen and antibody.
4. The conformation of antigen and antibody is critical to the precise spatial configurations between active sites.
5. Binding occurs through numerous reversible noncovalent interactions.
6. There is reaction ratio freedom in antigen-antibody union and aggregation.
7. Antisera contain a wide variety of antibodies, from several clones of lymphocytes, toward different antigenic determinants.
8. Each antibody in an antiserum demonstrates a variation in binding characteristics.

ANTIBODY SPECIFICITY AND AFFINITY

The specificity and affinity of antibody for antigen is confusing owing to the heterogeneity of antisera and the multivalency of antigen. By studying the reaction of antibody to hapten, it becomes possible to clarify basic principles. The reaction of hapten with antibody is a reaction in which a single determinant is attracted to and bound at a single binding site. In equation 4-7, the rate of association is expressed as k_1.

$$Hp + Ab \xrightarrow{k_1} HpAb \qquad \text{(Eq. 4-7)}$$

The rate of association depends on the unique characteristics of both molecules as determined by the sum of the effects of the interatomic interactions, hydrophobicity, and steric relationships. Equation 4-8 describes k_2, the dissociation constant. This constant is an expression of the rate at which the complex dissociates.

$$HpAb \xrightarrow{k_2} Hp + Ab \qquad \text{(Eq. 4-8)}$$

The dissociation constant indicates the avidity of the complex. The slower the rate of dissociation the more avid the complex. Avidity expresses the strength of bonds already formed. Often immunologists look at k_1 as affinity, the attraction of both molecules to each other. The combined equation 4-9 defines the total reversible reaction kinetics.

$$Hp + Ab \underset{k_2}{\overset{k_1}{\rightleftarrows}} HpAb \qquad \text{(Eq. 4-9)}$$

Through mathematical manipulation of equation 4-9, as shown in equations 4-10 and 4-11, it is possible to derive K, the intrinsic affinity constant.

$$k_1\,[Hp]\,[Ab] \rightleftarrows [HpAb]\,k_2 \qquad \text{(Eq. 4-10)}$$

$$\frac{[Hp]\,[Ab]}{[HpAb]} = \frac{k_2}{k_1} = K \qquad \text{(Eq. 4-11)}$$

If one measures any two parameters of equation 4-9 when the reaction is at equilibrium, it is possible to calculate K. The bracketed terms indicate equilibrium molar concentrations. A verbal description of K follows: The affinity constant, K, is the reciprocal of the free hapten where half the available antibody sites are bound. If K is equal to 4×10^5 liter/mole, it would indicate that at a free hapten concentration of 4×10^{-5} M one-half the antibody-binding sites are filled. If we had an antibody with a higher avidity and affinity, then the hapten would be more rapidly attracted to the antibody site and dissociate more slowly from the binding site. Therefore a much lower free hapten concentration could be reached and still bind half of the sites. Hence a K of 1×10^9 liter/mole would signify that one-half the sites are filled at a free hapten concentration of 1×10^{-9} M.

Affinity constants also allow an assessment of avidity and specificity. Avid antibodies have a high average affinity constant, K. In newer immunoassays we make use of hapten-antibody reactions. However, we more frequently use a heterologous antisera directed at multivalent antigens. In this situation avidity is greater than the sum of the strength of individual bonds. As seen in Fig. 4-9, an IgM directed against a polyvalent antigen derives a bonus effect, a sharp rise in

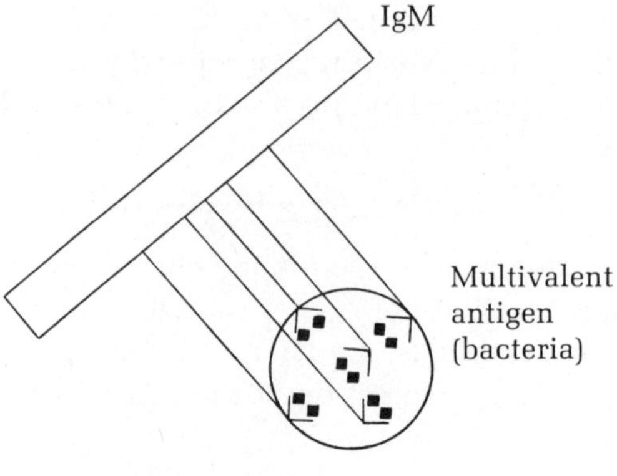

Bonus effect

Fig. 4-9. Binding of IgM to multivalent antigen (bacteria) results in greater binding strength than the sum of each Fab binding strength (bonus effect).

Table 11. Demonstrate the manipulation of data on three antisera that were titrated against the same antigen

	1:2	1:4	1:8	1:16	1:64
A	++ ++	++ ++	++	++	0
B	++	++	+	+	0
C	++	++	++	++	0

avidity. A great deal of information about an antiserum can be obtained via serial dilution. The antiserum is diluted serially and equal amounts of antigen are added to each tube. The end point or the last tube showing a reaction is the titer, usually expressed as the reciprocal of the dilution. As shown in Table 11, if an attempt is made to assess the amount of reaction in each, one can estimate avidity. The higher the total (individual evaluations 1+ to 4+) the more avid the antibody.

Note that in the data shown in Table 11, all three antisera have a titer of 1 : 16. If we add the semiquantitative evaluations of each reaction, we would find that "A" has an avidity quotient of 11, while "B" has an avidity quotient of 6, and "C" a quotient of 8. Antiserum "A" is more avid than "B" or "C".

The degree of cross-reactivity that antisera display can be critical to any immunoassay. Cross-reactivity is the opposite of specificity and indicates the capacity of the antisera to distinguish between homologous and heterologous antigens. Evaluation of affinity constants provides an excellent means to assess specificity or cross-reactivity. If the affinity constants of antisera for various antigens are known, then a single general rule will provide the means to evaluate specificity. The greater the difference in affinities between an antiserum and two antigens, the less cross-reactivity will be seen. Conversely, the closer the affinities of an antibody for two antigens, the more likely cross-reactivity will be observed. This concept can be misleading for it seems to say that an extremely high affinity reaction will be very specific. An antibody-antigen reaction with a high affinity constant will tend to bind structurally related antigens more strongly than would a lower affinity constant antibody. The decision to use a particular antisera in an assay can be looked at carefully from several points of view. However, the final criterion frequently is a practical evaluation involving "trial and error"; for economy titer is an important function, but the role of affinity, avidity and specificity in the choice of antisera cannot be forgotten.

ENVIRONMENTAL INFLUENCES ON ANTIGEN-ANTIBODY REACTIONS

Temperature

As mentioned, k_1, the rate of association of antigen and antibody, is extremely fast. A major rate-limiting factor for union appears to be temperature. Temperature exerts its effect in several ways. The most basic effect is manifested through diffusion. The rate of diffusion increases with increases in temperature, and therefore one would expect k_1 to increase in all reactions where temperature increases until a finite point where denaturation of reactants occurs. However, when many reactions are followed at temperatures ranging from 0° C to 40° C, the results are far more unpredictable than expected. The reaction of certain antibodies with antigens results in the formation of a more stable complex and the release of considerable energy, antibodies of the IgM class for example. These energy-releasing reactions are enhanced by cold temperatures and are termed "exothermic reactions." At higher temperatures the complex appears to absorb energy that inhibits the release of energy resulting in dissociation. Conversely, a second group of antibodies, warm-acting antibodies, are considered endothermic. These warm-acting antibodies require heat and energy to form stable complexes with antigens. Colder temperatures are incapable of supplying sufficient energy and in turn slow association. Temperatures above 40° C affect the conformation of antibody and antigen. As seen earlier, this denaturing process may lead to loss of all activity. As the temperature increases, enough energy is supplied to decrease the stability of the immune complex and enhance dissociation.

Salt concentration

Studies to clarify the effect of salt concentration on the rate of association of antigen and antibody have been difficult to interpret. Low salt concentrations aid antigen binding. Salt primarily exerts its effect through the ionic strength of the media. At low ionic strengths, the maximum number of ionic groups would be available at the active sites for binding between antigen and antibody. It would appear, then, that at low salt concentrations one would enhance association. In fact, at low ionic strength the immune reaction is in a precarious environment. At low salt concentrations nonspecific precipitation of euglobulins occurs. This salting out of antibody at low salt concentrations is manifested via a loss of activity. At high ionic strength of high salt concentrations the ionic groupings at the active sites of antigen and antibody are neutralized. The loss of these groups inhibits binding and causes a marked reduction in affinity. The dilution of serum for analysis via immunoassay is a major source of technical error. Any dilution must be such that the final sample has an ionic strength that is very close to that in the original sample.

pH

The presence of many disulfide bonds in the antibody molecule makes antibodies remarkably stable to pH changes. However, pH change does affect activity. Primarily, changes in hydrogen ion concentration affect activity through the so-called protonic effect of amino acids. Changes in ionization occur over a range of pH variations (Chapter 1). The resultant changes in ionization have two outcomes. First, changes in ionization may lead to conformational changes in antigen, antibody, or both. Second, changes in pH lead to modification of affinity due to changes that occur at critical binding ionization groups (Chapters 1 and 2).

Concentration of reactants

In the initial stages of research and development of most assays a cross-titration is required. This titration, as seen in Table 12, involves the serial dilution of antigen and antibody. An aliquot of each dilution of antigen is allowed to react with every dilution of antibody. One can evaluate the effect of zonal phenomena and choose the appropriate dilution of both reactants for use in the assay. Diffusion, as already mentioned, can be a rate-limiting factor in the immunoreaction.

Table 12. Cross-titration to establish optimum concentrations of antigen and antibody

				Ag		
		1:2	**1:4**	**1:8**	**1:16**	**1:32**
	1:2	−	−	−	−	−
	1:4	−	±	−	−	−
	1:8	−	+	+	−	−
Ab	1:16	−	+	+	−	−
	1:32	−	±	−	−	−
	1:64	−	−	−	−	−

High dilutions of both antigen and antibody, although at equivalence, may increase diffusion distance and may appear to inhibit union. The callous handling of serum samples, antisera, and/or antigen preparations will surely result in erroneous and misleading data. Reactant concentration, pH, ionic strength, and temperature are the most frequently abused reaction parameters. However, these environmental factors are far from all the interferences encountered in the performance of immunoassays. There exist many non-specific interferences that common sense should eliminate. Particular substances and critical environments for specific clinical assays will be reviewed under each assay.

READINGS AND RESOURCES

Chase, M. W., and Williams, C. A., editors: Methods in immunology immunochemistry, vols. 1 to 3, New York, 1967-1971, Academic Press, Inc.

Heidelberger, M.: Quantitative absolute methods in the study of and antibody reactions, Bacteriol. Rev. **3**:49, 1949.

Haurowitz, F.: Immunochemistry and the biosynthesis of antibodies, New York, 1968, John Wiley & Sons, Inc.

Hughes-Jones, N. C.: The nature of the reaction of antigen with antibody, Br. Med. Bull. **19**:3, 1963.

Kabat, E. A.: Kabat and Meyer's experimental immunochemistry, ed. 2, Springfield, Ill., 1961, Charles C Thomas, Publisher.

Landsteiner, K.: The specificity of serological reactions, Cambridge, Mass., 1945, Harvard University Press.

Nezlin, R. S.: Biochemistry of antibodies, New York, 1970, Plenum Press, Inc.

SECTION TWO

IMMUNODIAGNOSTIC TECHNIQUES

Historically, immunology has had an important role in research and medicine. Great advances in immunization against polio, rabies, and diphtheria are but a few examples of these strides. Interest in diagnosing venereal disease provided the greatest impetus to the development of immunodiagnostic technique. In the clinical laboratory, serology was synonymous with immunology. Laboratories were primarily concerned with the detection of antibodies, the telltale signs of infection, and serologic identification of putative microorganisms.

Today laboratorians still search for the trails left by man's response to pathogenic organisms. However, now immunologists look for antibodies against a wide variety of infectious organisms including bacteria, parasites, fungi, and viruses. A laboratory devoted to immunochemistry or immunodiagnostics has a new mission. It is concerned with the detection and quantitation of clinically significant antigens and antibodies. The sensitivity and specificity of immunoassays allows not only the detection of antibodies to pathogenic organisms but the identification of the organism itself. Further, these assays provide the means to quantitate the blood level of drugs used to treat the infection. Advances in immunodiagnostics (presently a more relevant name than serology) have indeed provided the stimulus and the means for parallel advances in science and medicine.

The second section of this book classifies in vitro immunoassays into the following categories: (1) precipitin tests, (2) agglutinin tests, (3) complement-employing assays, (4) neutralization tests, and (5) assays utilizing labeled antigens and/or antibodies. The purpose of this classification is to develop test type generalizations prior to the investigation of specific assays. The overall objectives of this second section are to clarify concepts, principles, methods, and interpretations of in vitro assays.

CHAPTER 5

Precipitin assays

The reaction of soluble antigens with antibodies may lead to the visible precipitation of the reactants. This precipitation develops because of the increased number of hydrophobic groups brought into close association with each other. When the number of hydrophobic groups reaches some critical level, the complex is able to effectively exclude water, hence to precipitate. Precipitation can then be considered a reaction that transforms soluble reactants into insoluble products. The precipitation reaction is the basic mechanism in a wide variety of immunoassays currently used in the clinical laboratory. Agar gel precipitin tests have enjoyed the greatest popularity over recent years. The simplicity of these assays surely is a factor in their popularity, but simplicity is not the major reason for the success of these tests. Precipitin assays combine method simplicity with excellent sensitivity and versatility. This chapter will be concerned with elucidating basic principles of precipitation.

As discussed earlier, union of antigen and antibody is the first step of precipitation. This step is rapid and is governed primarily by:

1. Van der Waals forces
2. Hydrogen bonding
3. Hydrophobic and hydrophilic interaction

The development of lattice formation from the immune complex is dependent on these factors and new variables.

1. Ratio of antigen to antibody
2. Salt concentration
3. pH
4. Temperature
5. Absolute concentrations of antigens and antibodies
6. Valence of antigens
7. Affinity of antigen for antibody

The factors listed above may act to enhance or inhibit lattice formation and therefore are critical to precipitation reactions.

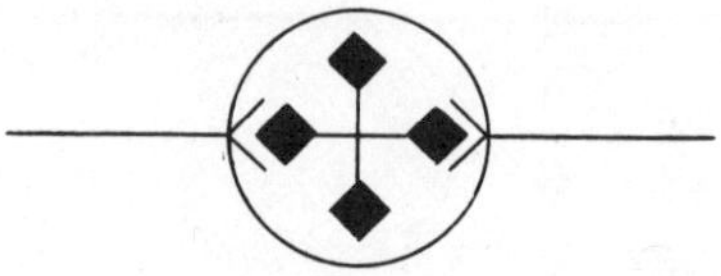

Fig. 5-1. Hypothetical univalent antibodies reacting with tetravalent antigen. Note open end of antibody symbol indicates lack of binding site.

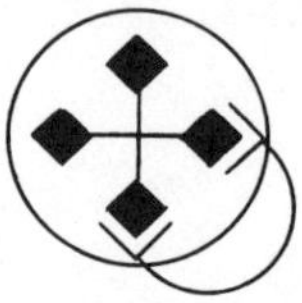

Fig. 5-2. Schematic representation of monogamous binding of two Fab sites of single antibody to separate antigenic determinants within single molecule or particle.

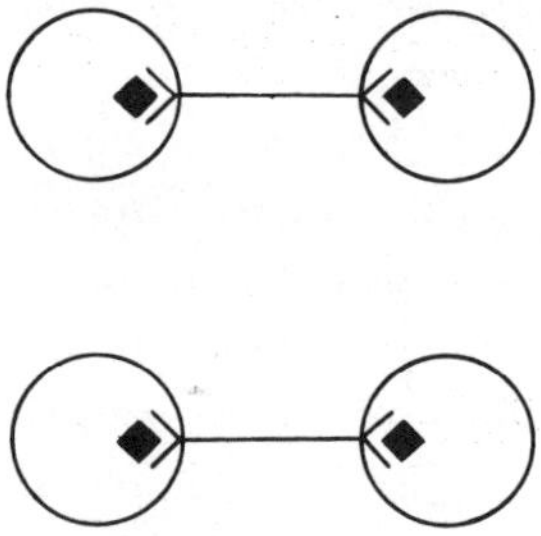

Fig. 5-3. Lattice formation inhibition owing to univalency of hapten or antigen. Note that it is unlikely that binding of two Fab sites could occur at the same moment to a single antigen determinant.

Some antibodies appear to be incapable of precipitation with antigen, and it was proposed by some researchers that these antibodies were univalent. As shown in Fig. 5-1, this theory speculated that a univalent antibody would have but one combining site (Fab). This univalent antibody clearly would be incapable of lattice formation as discussed in Chapter 4. Although this was a logical explanation, it was a false one. No proof has ever been shown to back up the presence of a naturally occurring univalent antibody. Current theories to explain this functional univalency, in some reactions, include the following: (1) If affinity of antigen for antibody is too low, it would allow dissociation to be as rapid as association and hinder precipitation. (2) If divalent antibody bound to two antigenic sites on a single antigen molecule, then the antibody would have no unbound Fab fragments to attack separate antigens (Fig. 5-2). (3) If the ligand were a univalent hapten or antigen, lattice formation would again be inhibited (Fig. 5-3). Precipitation assays are remarkably effected by zonal phenomena. If optimal concentrations of antigen and antibody are mixed together, precipitation occurs. However, the addition of excess antigen or antibody to the precipitate results in the formation of soluble complexes and the transformation of the insoluble precipitate to a soluble form.

INTERFACIAL RING TEST

The interfacial test offers a rapid means to detect soluble antigen or antibody. The antigen solution is overlaid onto the antibody solution. This can be accomplished in any size test tube or even capillary tubes. Antigen diffuses down into the antibody layer forming a concentration gradient. When the optimum antigen-antibody ratio exists, a sharp precipitin band forms. Any factor that increases opacity of either solution may interfere with the visual interpretation, for example, lipemia. In 1930 it was noted that patients with pneumococcal pneumonia developed a reactive protein. This protein was capable of precipitating the somatic C-polysaccharide of the pneumococcus organism. Early workers felt that this protein was an antibody that could prove valuble in aiding the diagnosis of pneumonia. It was later shown *not* to be an immunoglobulin and its presence was noted in a variety of inflammatory states.

C-reactive protein (CRP) is heat labile and appears rapidly after the onset of illness. For this reason it is referred to as an acute-phase protein. The major value of CRP is as an aid in evaluating the efficiency of a particular treatment. Owing to the abrupt nature of this acute-phase protein, when proper treatment is initiated CRP rapidly disappears from the serum.

Principle. Purified CRP is strongly immunogenic in rabbits. Animal immunization provides the clinical laboratory with a potent antisera capable of precipitating CRP. This antiserum is used in several immunoassays, most notably the capillary precipitation tests, gel diffusion test, latex agglutination tests, and recently, radioimmunoassays. Capillary precipitation can be accomplished one of two ways. The first makes use of the ability of CRP to selectively precipitate C-polysaccharide, and the second makes use of antibody specificity for CRP (Fig. 5-4). In Fig. 5-4, *A,* a ring will form at the interface between serum containing CRP and the purified C-polysaccharide. In Fig. 5-4, *B,* serum and anti-CRP are

Prevalence of CRP in various disorders

Consistently found in	Less consistently found in
Bacterial infections	Active rheumatoid arthritis
Active rheumatic fever	Systemic lupus erythematosus
Acute myocardial infarction	Viral infections
Malignant diseases	Tuberculosis

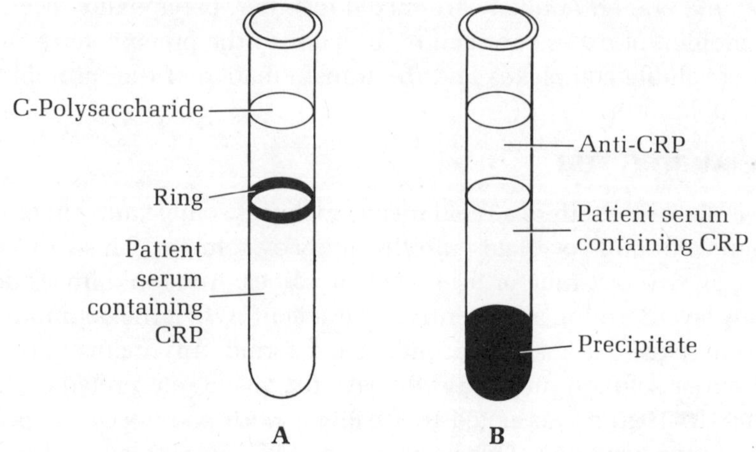

Fig. 5-4. Depicts two alternative approaches to capillary precipitin tests for C-reactive protein. **A,** Utilizes purified C-polysaccharide laid carefully over patient sample with precipitation occurring at interface with CRP-positive patient serum. **B,** Utilizes anti-CRP to precipitate patient CRP.

mixed and the precipitation settles to the bottom of the capillary tube. Either ring size or the amount of precipitation can be graded semiquantitatively.

Interpretation. As shown in the boxed material on p. 69, CRP is almost always found in certain infectious diseases and in many noninfectious inflammatory conditions. Indeed the problem with CRP is that the test is too sensitive and therefore lacks specificity.

SINGLE DIFFUSION–ONE DIMENSION ASSAY

In 1946 Oudin developed the single diffusion–one dimension agar precipitin assay. This step in the development of immunoassays in gel was an important step for clinical immunology. The procedure involves heating agar and allowing it to melt and then cooling it to 50° C. At this temperature agar remains fluid, yet antibody is not destroyed. The antiserum is mixed with the liquid agar and poured into tubes. The antigen solution is laid over the cooled agar. Antigen alone diffuses, hence single diffusion in only one dimension—down.

The method used by Oudin was modified many times. The first major modification was to substitute 1.5% agarose for agar. Agarose is impermeable to substances with a molecular weight greater than 200,000 daltons. This feature allows the diffusion of antigen but immobilizes the immune complex. The main principles of all immunogel assays were developed in Oudin's assay. As antigen diffuses into the agar, a concentration gradient is formed, the front, containing the lowest concentration. Diffusion continues until the optimum antigen-antibody ratio is reached; at that point precipitation develops. If antigen continues to move down into the agar, the optimum ratio is disturbed. This postzone results in solubilization of the precipitate. The reversibility of the reaction promotes continued diffusion. Migration of the band will persist until there exists an optimum ratio of antigen to antibody and depletion of the free antigen gradient. Simple reasoning should allow the elucidation of those factors that govern the movement of this band. The most obvious is zonal phenomena. The sequence of equivalence—postzone, equivalence, postzone—is surely a key factor in the band migration. What governs the distance of band migration? As we have seen, the depletion of the moving free antigen front will surely halt band movement. Therefore a critical factor in distance of band movement is antigen concentration. Another not so obvious variable is the diffusion coefficient of the antigen. This coefficient is derived mathematically from the molecular weight and shape of the antigen molecule. Basically, the lower the molecular weight the faster the rate of diffusion. Countering this size-rate factor is the effect of antigen shape. If the antigen is large and bulky, diffusion will be slowed. The distance of band migration is also related to time and the type, quality, and concentration of antibody in agar. Distance of band migration is proportional to the square of time. If all antigen is consumed in complex formation, then migration ceases; hence the antibody concentration in agarose is an important factor. If the antibody concentration is very high in agar, then the band will not migrate far. Clearly a low-affinity reaction will act to inhibit band formation; therefore the choice of the animal system to prepare the precipitating antisera may also be an important factor. The classical assay results in the formation of a precipitate band forming for each distinct pair of immune partners, and each band will migrate uniquely depending on the factors mentioned. The assay is ideal for detecting precipitating antibodies and for determining the minimum number of immune systems. There are two major limitations that hinder the clinical usefulness of this assay. First, it is very difficult to accurately quantitate antigen. Second, it is even more difficult to identify the specific bands of interest among the array that might be present. The assay cannot be conveniently used with nonprecipitating antibodies.

The following hypothetical assay will serve to reinforce some of the basic concepts in gel diffusion and particularly in the Oudin assay. A heterologous antiserum prepared in rabbit against pooled human serum is dispersed in agar. This study will attempt to quantitate IgM using Oudin's assay as described previously and seen in Fig. 5-5. In separate tubes the immunogel is overlaid with two purified standards, IgM and IgG. The third tube is overlaid with the patient sample and the fourth with a control. The assumption we would like to make is basic. If the patient's IgM band migrates further than the standard, it can be assumed that the patient's IgM is greater in concentration. This must be true because all other variables for the migrating distance are equal. To aid quality control a fourth tube would be overlaid with a control serum with known IgG and IgM concentrations. In tube number 1 (Fig. 5-5) IgM, now the antigen, would diffuse into the agar. Its high molecular weight would tend to decrease diffusion rate, while this rate would be tempered by its bulky shape. IgG, in tube 2, has a much lower molecu-

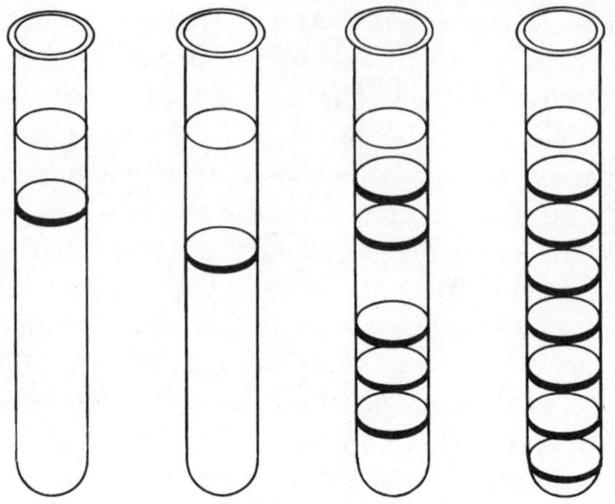

Fig. 5-5. Hypothetical assay using the methodology of Oudin to estimate IgG and IgM in patient serum. All four tubes contain an antihuman serum immunogel; tube No. **1** is overlaid with purified IgM standard, tube No. **2** is overlaid with purified IgG standard, tube No. **3** is overlaid with patient serum, and tube No. **4** is overlaid with control serum. Note multiple bands in tube Nos. **3** and **4. 1,** IgM; **2,** IgG; **3,** patient; **4,** control.

lar weight and would tend to diffuse rapidly; the small shape enhances diffusion and each particular physical characteristic aids in developing a unique diffusion constant for each immunoglobulin. It is most useful to choose standards with antigen concentrations close to that of a normal adult mean, 1200 mg/dl IgG and 125 mg/dl IgM. The titer of the antisera in agar would be critical; too high a titer may inhibit diffusion while too low a titer may promote the formation of complexes but inhibit precipitation. In tubes 1 and 2 primary factor governing band migration is antigen concentration. Now a mere comparison with the appropriate band in tubes 3 and 4 should provide the answer to what the concentrations are in the patient and control samples. However, when one inspects tubes 3 and 4, the problem is evident. There exist approximately 50 bands in the reaction of antihuman sera with human sera. Which band is IgG and which is IgM? It would be very difficult to compare and identify the bands in the reference standard with the bands seen in the patient's serum. If we used monospecific antiserum in agar, would this solve the problem? Purified μ heavy chains are isolated and used to immunize rabbits to prepare an anti-IgM antiserum. This antiserum is absorbed with pooled human serum depleted of IgM to further increase antiserum specificity and is then used in the following manner. Paired tubes are set up as in Fig. 5-6. The immunogel is overlaid with IgM reference standard in tube 1 and patient's serum in tube 2. Since the same antibody is used in both tubes and the time and temperature are determined in advance, all parameters except IgM concentration are fixed. On completion of the test time one band is found in

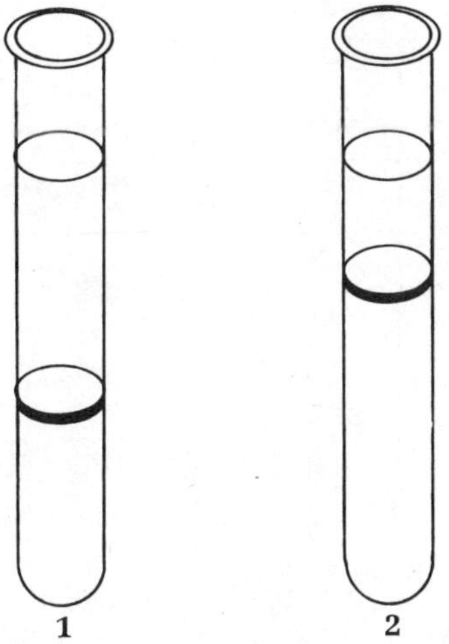

Fig. 5-6. Oudin's assay using monospecific anti-IgM in gel tube No. **1** is overlaid with normal reference standard, while tube No. **2** is patient sample. Distance traversed by patient IgM is approximately half distance of reference standard IgM migration. **1,** IgM reference. **2,** Patient sample.

each tube and a comparison of distance gives relative information about the patient's IgM serum level. In inspecting the patient tube several possibilities might exist. One possibility would be the finding of no bands at all. This could indicate a deficiency in the patient. Absence of band formation may be due to prozone or postzone. Another possibility is the presence of several bands. Intuitively this indicates more than one antigen-antibody system. However our antisera is μ chain specific. Assuming that the antisera were properly absorbed, we are left with one conclusion, polymeric IgM. If the patient sample had 7S, 19S, and 23S IgM present, then the migration of the three forms would be influenced by their size and shape along with concentration, resulting in the formation of several bands. Occasionally, antigens adsorb to each other forming a nondiffusing globule, clearly a source of error. If the patient's sample is reduced or denatured, there exists the possibility that free μ chains could confuse the above assay. Lipemia or hemolysis may obstruct identification of precipitin bands or appear to be a band. This problem necessitates sampling blood when the patient is in the preabsorptive (fasting) state. These principles and concepts developed in Oudin's single diffusion–one dimension assay are relevant to the currently used agar gel techniques of today.

In reality, the double diffusion–one dimension assay is but a minor modification of Oudin's system. In the double diffusion–one dimension assay the immunoagar is overlaid with clear agar, which in turn is overlaid with antigen. Both the antigen and the antibody diffuse into the neutral zone. The fronts meet and

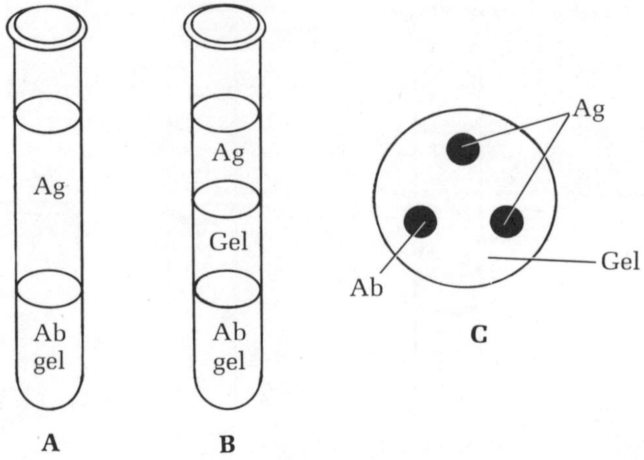

Fig. 5-7. Typical arrangements of gel diffusion immunoassays. **A,** Oudin's single diffusion–one dimension with antigen solution overlaid onto immunogel. **B,** Double diffusion–one dimension assay with antigen solution and antibody gel separated by neutral gel. **C,** Ouchterlöny's double diffusion–two dimension assay with antigen solutions in separate precut agar well and antiserum in precut well.

finally optimum concentrations are attained, resulting in the formation of precipitin bands. If antigen is in excess of antibody, the band moves toward the antibody zone, and the reverse occurs if antibody is in excess (Fig. 5-7, *B*). The double diffusion–one dimension assay was the basic assay Ouchterlöny used in developing the elegant system that bears his name.

OUCHTERLÖNY'S DOUBLE DIFFUSION IN TWO DIMENSIONS

Ouchterlöny placed antigen and antibody in separate wells cut out of neutral agar in Petri dishes. He found that antigen and antibody diffused into the neutral agar and the fronts formed precipitin bands at Ag/Ab equivalence. If antigen was in excess, solubilization of the precipitate resulted in apparent movement of the band closer to the antibody well. Although diffusion occurs radially from the well, the precipitin bands appear as arcs between the antigen and antibody wells. The precipitin arc is specifically impermeable to homologous antibody and antigen, allowing nonrelated immune complexes to pass through the band but acting as a barrier or sink to all similar complexes. The diffusion of both immune partners is governed by the same factors discussed earlier—molecular weight, shape, concentration of antigen and antibody, and so on.

The choice of well arrangement depends on the objective of the assay. The configuration used in Fig. 5-9 is ideal for comparing two antigens. Once precipitation occurs, the density of the precipitate increases with time. As shown in Fig. 5-8, fusion of precipitin lines occurs when both antigens are identical. Antigens in well 1 and 2, because they are identical, diffuse radially at equivalent rates.

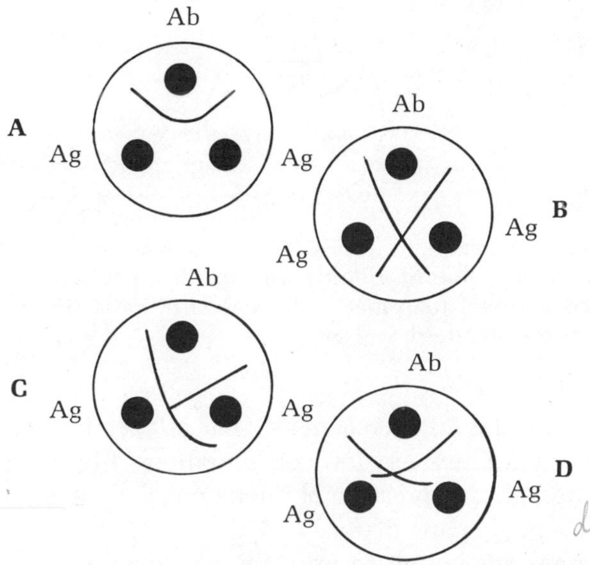

Fig. 5-8. Basic Ouchterlöny well configurations and reactions when evaluating two antigens tested against single antiserum. Reaction **A** is one of identity, while reaction **B** is nonidentity, **C** is partial identity, and **D** is double partial identity.

Antibody diffuses out of well 3 radially, and the arcs between wells 1 and 3 and 2 and 3 fuse. Fusion occurs because all variables governing diffusion are equal for antigen 1 and 2, and the band forms an immunospecific barrier. On the other hand, if they are totally unrelated, diffusion rates vary and precipitin arcs do not act as barriers for the unrelated antigen. In the reaction of nonidentity the two bands form an X or cross (Fig. 5-8, *B*). A third basic reaction (Fig. 5-8, *C*), is that of partial identity. Fusion of bands with the development of a characteristic spur indicates partial identity. Partial identity would be seen if antigen 1 was human albumin while antigen 2 was simian albumin and the antibody was antihuman albumin. The spur extends toward the cross-reacting antigen, in the above example toward the simian albumin. An occasional source of error is shown in Fig. 5-8, *D*, double partial identity. Reactions of nonidentity must be examined carefully for easily missed attenuation and curvature of the double spur. Clinically, Ouchterlöny's immunogel assay has been used for the analysis of a variety of antigens, including viral, bacterial, endocrine, and cancer-associated antigens.

Alpha-fetoprotein (AFP)

Alpha-fetoprotein (AFP) is an α_1-globulin and is glycoprotein in nature. AFP has a molecular weight of approximately 65,000 to 70,000 and is synthesized normally in fetal liver and yolk sac. The biologic function of AFP is unknown. The blood level peaks 13 to 15 weeks postconception and drops to the adult nor-

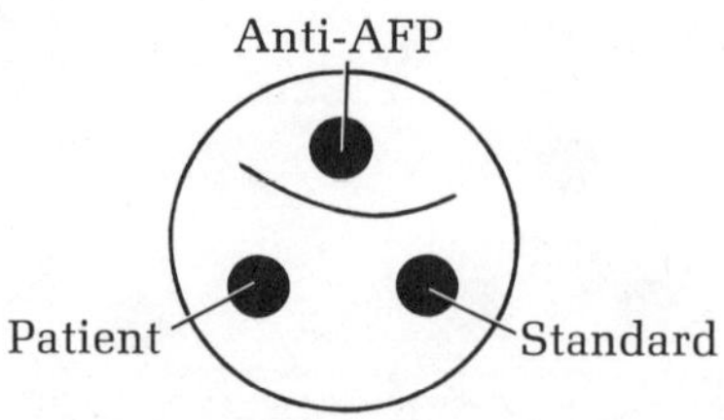

Fig. 5-9. Ouchterlöny reaction for alpha-fetoprotein assay. Note that patient sample front formed a precipitin line of identity with the AFP precipitin band. Patient band migration distance is longer than that of the standard, indicating concentration levels higher than that of the standard.

mal, 1 ng/ml, before the infant reaches 1 year of age. This protein is normally present in the blood at these very low concentrations. Elevations occur in serum AFP, probably through derepression of a fetal-phase gene, in certain neoplastic disorders and in some hepatic diseases.

Principle. The normal adult serum AFP is below the sensitivity of agar diffusion techniques. Therefore it is possible to use Ouchterlöny's gel technique to screen patient serum in search for identity with purified AFP. Identification of AFP indicates blood levels that can be detected by gel diffusion, hence an elevation above normal.

Methodology. As shown in Fig. 5-9, anti-AFP challenges an AFP standard and a patient's sera. The agar plate is incubated in a cool moist chamber at least 24 hours. (Longer time usually results in denser bands.)

Interpretation. Lines of identity with patient's serum and purified AFP indicate the presence of AFP in abnormal concentrations in the patient sample. Comparison of positions of the standard and patients' arcs gives semiquantitative information about antigen concentration. AFP has been detected in 60% to 80% of the patients with hepatoma. Presence of AFP by agar diffusion may be a helpful diagnostic aid, quantitation of AFP by enzyme immunoassay or radioimunoassay must be used to follow the disease process. These latter discriminating assays have led to renewed interest in the diagnostic value of AFP.

IMMUNOELECTROPHORESIS (IEP)

Immunoelectrophoresis (IEP), developed by Grabar and Williams in 1953, is used to study antibodies and antigens. The IEP technique makes use of two properties of the molecule under study, the characteristic electrophoretic mobility (Chapter 1) and immunologic specificity detected in agar gel. Modifications of the basic technique have become clinically useful in screening serum for specific protein abnormalities, while semiquantitatively assessing the major protein fractions. The procedure involves electrophoretic separation of the antigen solution, commonly serum. Once fractioned, the antigens diffuse into agar and react with specific or multivalent antisera. As shown in Fig. 5-10, *A*, the serum, urine,

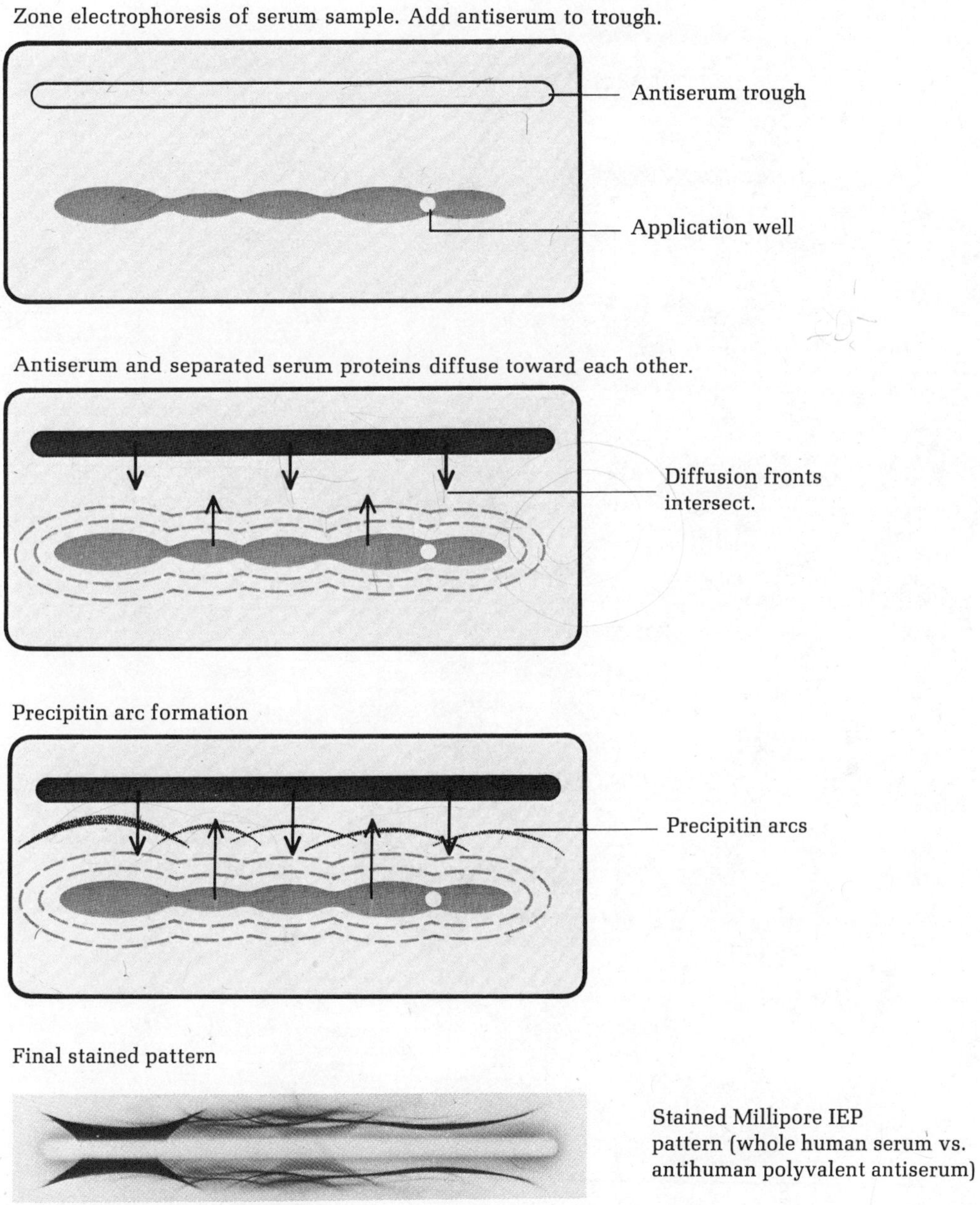

Fig. 5-10. Immunoelectrophoresis. (Reprinted with permission of Millipore Corporation, Bedford, Massachusetts.)

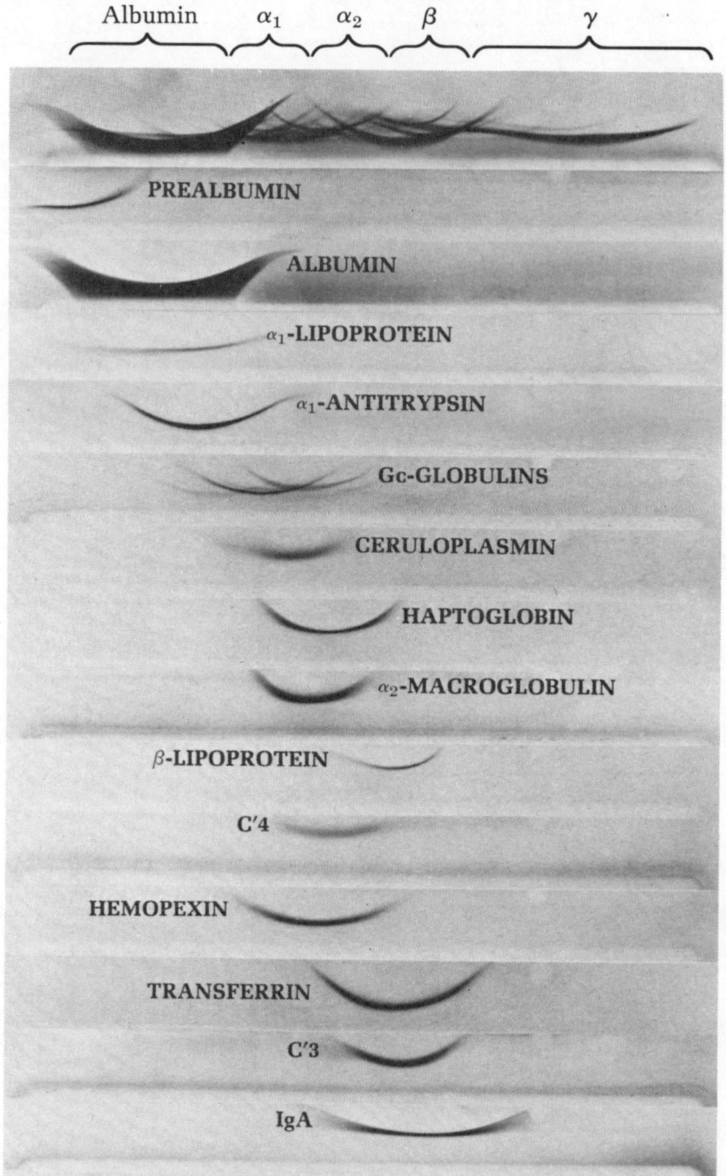

Fig. 5-11. Major precipitin arcs identifiable by immunoelectrophoresis. (Reprinted with permission of Millipore Corporation, Bedford, Massachusetts.)

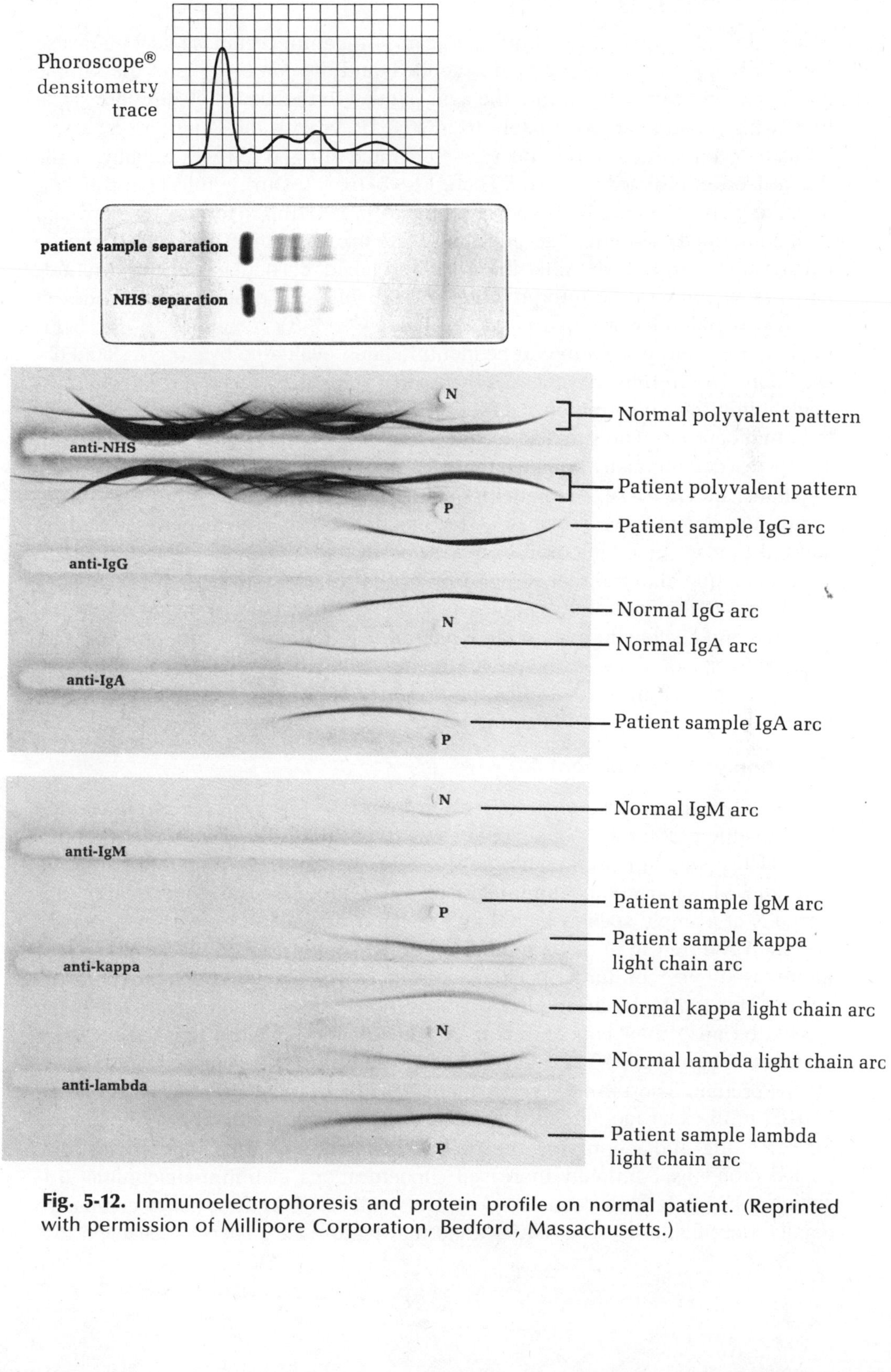

Fig. 5-12. Immunoelectrophoresis and protein profile on normal patient. (Reprinted with permission of Millipore Corporation, Bedford, Massachusetts.)

or spinal fluid is applied to a buffered agarose medium (cellulose acetate is also sometimes used). An electric field is applied, and the components of the sample are separated. A trough cut into the agar parallel to the axis of electrophoresis is filled with antisera (approximately 10 to 20 μl). As with the Ouchterlöny assay, diffusion occurs into the neutral agar. Separated antigen diffuses radially, while the antiserum diffuses as a band (note Fig. 5-10, *B*). During diffusion the agar must be incubated in a moist cool chamber. A precipitin arc forms between each antigen-antibody system. The location of the arc is furthest from the immune partner that is in excess. All of the rules developed, particularly in the Ouchterlöny assay, apply to the interpretation of IEP. One can easily interpret lines of identity, nonidentity, and partial identity (see Fig. 5-8). As shown in Fig. 5-11, the major protein precipitin can be identified and evaluated by simple visual observation. To carefully investigate critical arcs such as those produced by immunoglobulins, it is an extremely useful procedure to assay the patient along with alternating controls. The simplest technique involves employing a multiple trough agar plate (commercially available) with suitable areas for six antisera challenges. As shown in Fig. 5-12, the patient sample is alternated with a normal control sample in electrophoresis zones. After electrophoresis, the patient's serum is allowed to react by double diffusion with polyvalent and monospecific antisera. This technique allows direct comparison of the patient's arc with a normal control. In a way the control arcs appear to fuse with their comparable bands in the patient sample, allowing precise and accurate evaluation of serum proteins. Deviations in size or shape of the precipitin arcs indicate the presence of abnormal concentrations of antigens and/or the presence of abnormal proteins. Fig. 5-13 illustrates typical deviation encountered in IEP.

Detection of M component

Usually a sharp spike on protein electrophoresis in the beta or gamma region indicates the proliferation of a single clone of plasma cells (Fig. 5-14). This uncontrolled malignant proliferation of a single clone of cells produces excessive quantities of homogenous immunoglobulin. The protein or immunoglobulin produced is of a single species including class and subclass. These M components are often referred to as paraproteins. Although protein electrophoresis is commonly used to screen for monoclonal gammopathy, there are outstanding drawbacks. The most significant drawback is that monoclonal increases may be missed because their concentrations are low or they may be masked by other proteins. When "spikes" are noted, further analysis is needed for identification of this protein. The term "M component," indicating *m*alignant or *m*onoclonal, is used until exact identification is made. IEP offers a relatively easy technique for screening and identifying these abnormal increases in patients with suspected problems. Markedly increased concentrations of immunoglobulins, unbalanced kappa/lambda ratio, or excessive synthesis of light or heavy chains are readily identifiable by IEP. These abnormal features are seen as localized dis-

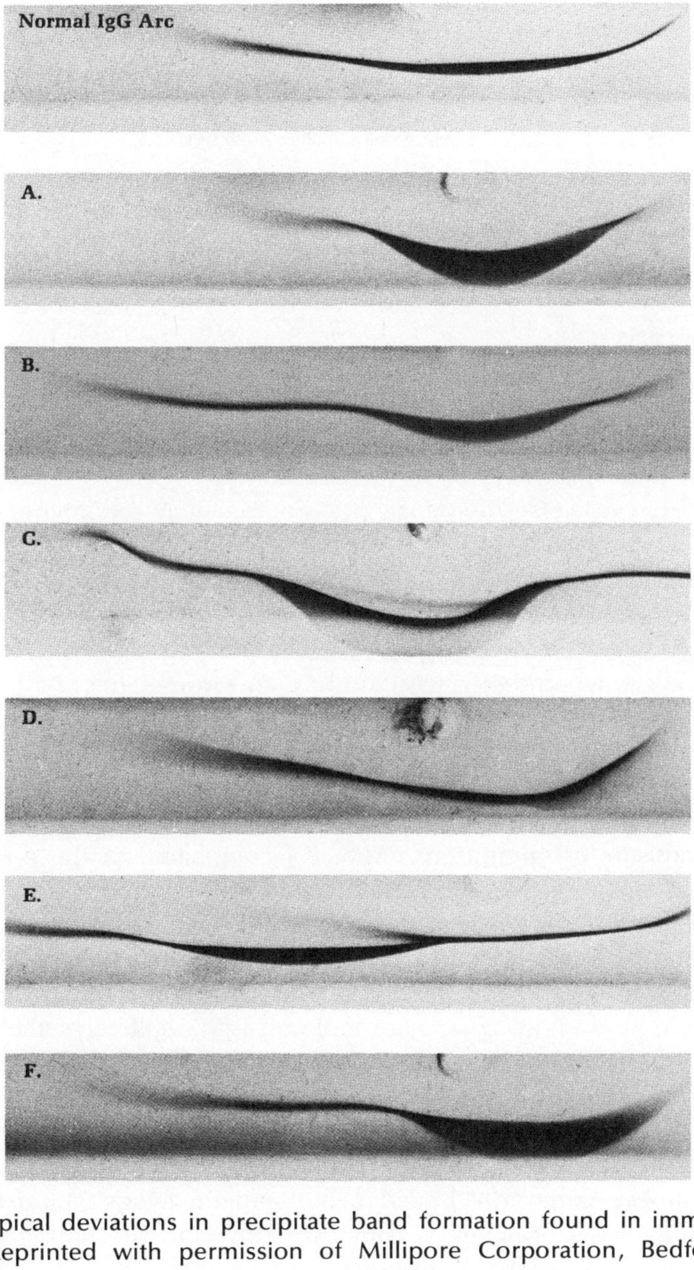

Fig. 5-13. Typical deviations in precipitate band formation found in immunoelectrophoresis. (Reprinted with permission of Millipore Corporation, Bedford, Massachusetts.)

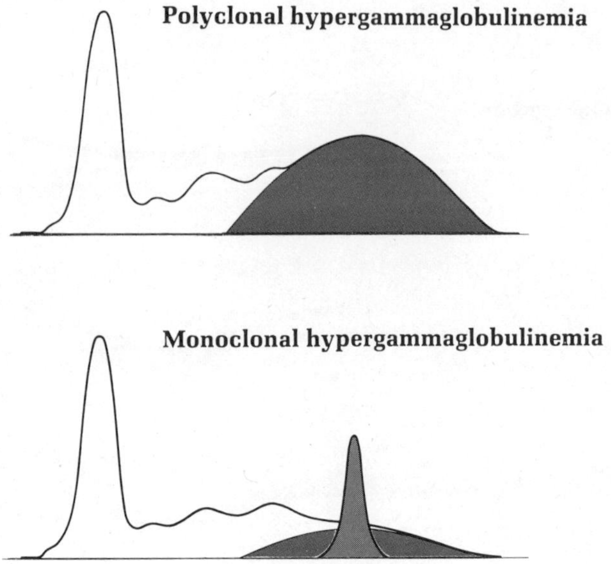

Fig. 5-14. Monoclonal versus polyclonal peaks on protein electrophoresis. (Reprinted with permission of Millipore Corporation, Bedford, Massachusetts.)

tortions or bulges when tested with antihuman serum. This first step is merely a means of screening for the presence of abnormality. The double diffusion reaction with specific antisera elaborates the final picture. Fig. 5-15 demonstrates a protein profile on a patient with an IgG (lambda) monoclonal gammopathy. Note that on protein electrophoresis an M component is seen. Upon IEP against polyvalent antisera a bulging arc is noted as compared to the normal human serum. When challenged with anti-IgG, the normal control produces the typical arc approximately in the midregion, between the well and trough. However, the patient serum, when tested with anti-IgG, results in an arc that is distorted and displaced. Prozone has forced the arc to shift close to the trough, indicating an excess of IgG. Analysis with anti-IgA and anti-IgM challenges shows relatively normal amounts of these proteins as does the anti-kappa challenge. When we look carefully at the anti-lambda reaction, we again see distortion and prozone. One must consider that in any monoclonal proliferation the serum would surely demonstrate an increase in only one type of light chain.

Methodology. As described previously the methodology includes:

1. Electrophoresis of patient serum and controls in alternating zones
2. Application of antisera to troughs
3. Incubation in moist chamber, approximately 24° C
4. Protein staining of precipitin arcs requiring deproteinization of all non-precipitated protein

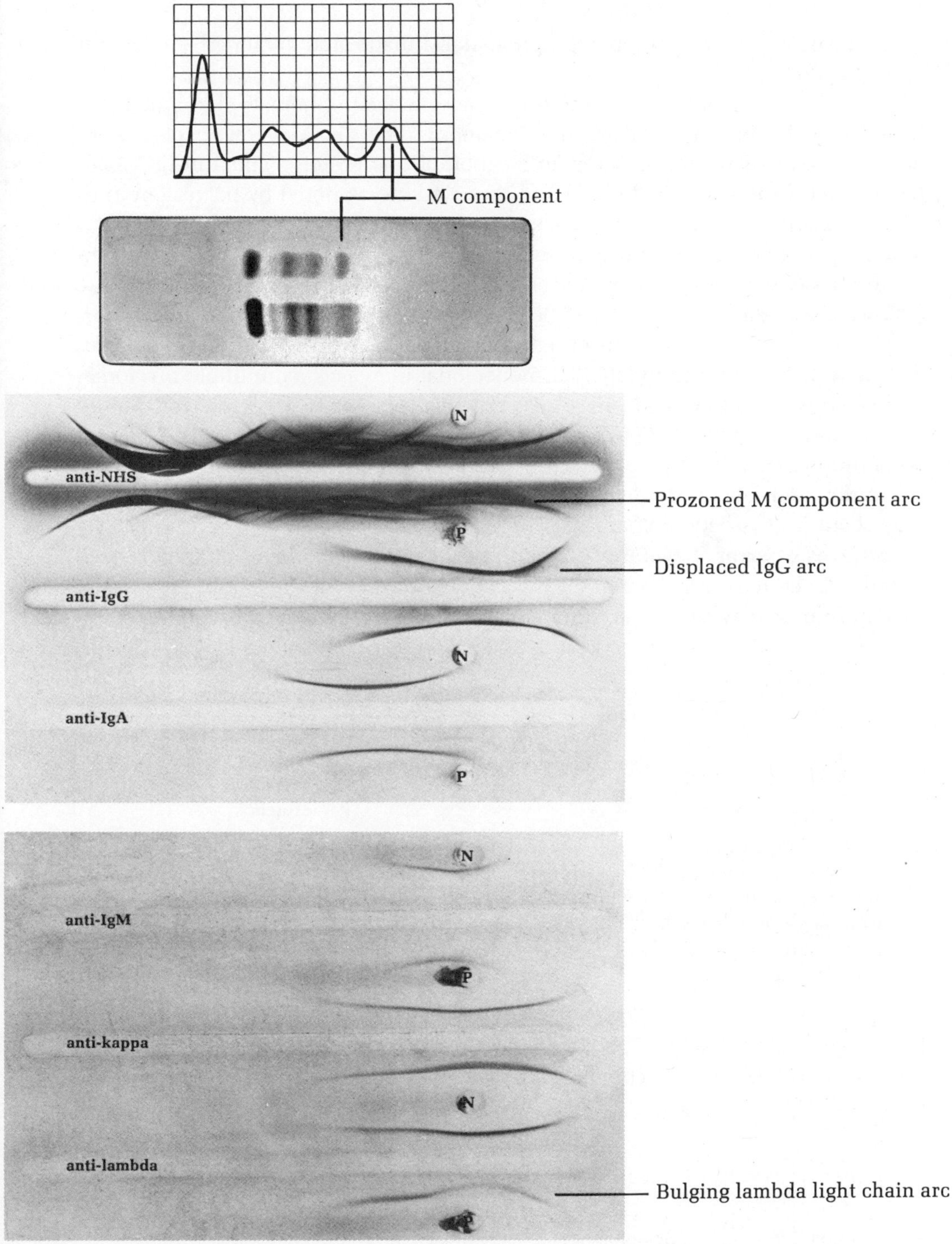

Fig. 5-15. Gammopathy profile on patient with an IgG lambda monoclonal gammopathy. (Reprinted with permission of Millipore Corporation, Bedford, Massachusetts.)

5. Visual observation (photograph usually made and included on patient report)

Interpretation. In Fig. 5-15 the initial protein electrophoresis alerts the technologist to the presence of an M component. The challenge with polyvalent antisera confirms the gamma region location of this protein. The anti-IgG challenge reveals the identical bulged and distorted arc as noted by polyvalent antisera. This anti-IgG reaction indicates that this abnormal protein is IgG and that it is in excess compared to the normal serum controls. The light chain antisera confirms the monoclonal character of this M component. This is revealed by the excessive lambda chain synthesis. Both IgM and IgA appear to be relatively normal. The unbalanced synthesis of light chains is the result of a single clone proliferation. It is tempting to label all monoclonal increases as multiple myeloma, a dreaded malignancy of plasma cells, but this represents a grave error. Monoclonal gammopathies are associated with a number of disorders, and the diagnosis of multiple myeloma rests with the diagnostician and the correlation of physical, x-ray, and laboratory data. The boxed material shows that a gammopathy may occur in a variety of conditions.

Sources of error. Several cautions in performing IEP should be emphasized in order to reduce error. Extremely high concentrations of the paraprotein in the patient sample may cause the formation of soluble complexes (postzone) leading

Malignancies of hematopoietic system*

Disease	Paraprotein
Multiple myeloma	IgG, IgA, IgD, IgE (kappa or lambda)
Macroglobulinemia (Waldenströms)	IgM (kappa or lambda)
Heavy chain disease (Franklin)	Fc fragment of IgG, IgA, or IgM
Cold agglutinin disease	IgM (kappa)
Bence Jones proteinemia	Kappa or lambda
Lymphoma	Kappa or lambda
Nonlymphoplasmacytic disorders	
Neoplasms, autoimmune diseases, chronic liver disease, chronic infections	IgG, IgA, IgM, IgD, or IgE (kappa or lambda)
Idiopathic/benign	
Apparently healthy subjects	IgG, IgA, IgM, IgD, or IgE (lambda or kappa)

*Modified from Immunoglobulin abnormality detection, Applications Monograph AM 310, Bedford, Mass., 1973, Millipore Corporation.

to an interpretation of hypoproteinemia. Postzone can also cause the arc to be closely associated with the antisera arc and may be missed. Some people feel that all patients' sera should be diluted 1:5 or 1:10 with saline solution prior to IEP to overcome this source of error. Antiserum specificity and potency can be checked by using carefully controlled assay parameters and comparing prior normal control assays with the present assay or periodic testing dilutions of antisera with normal controls. Other major sources of error in IEP include inpurities or imperfections in agarose, insufficient electrophoresis, unreliable antisera, poorly absorbed antisera, and excess antisera in trough or serum in electrophoresis zone. Immune complexes present in the serum of patients with systemic lupus erythematosus or rheumatoid arthritis may precipitate during electrophoresis and lead to erroneous results.

RADIAL IMMUNODIFFUSION (RID)

Serum proteins

Radial immunodiffusion (RID) remains the most popular of agar immunoassays. This single diffusion–two dimension assay is presently considered the refer-

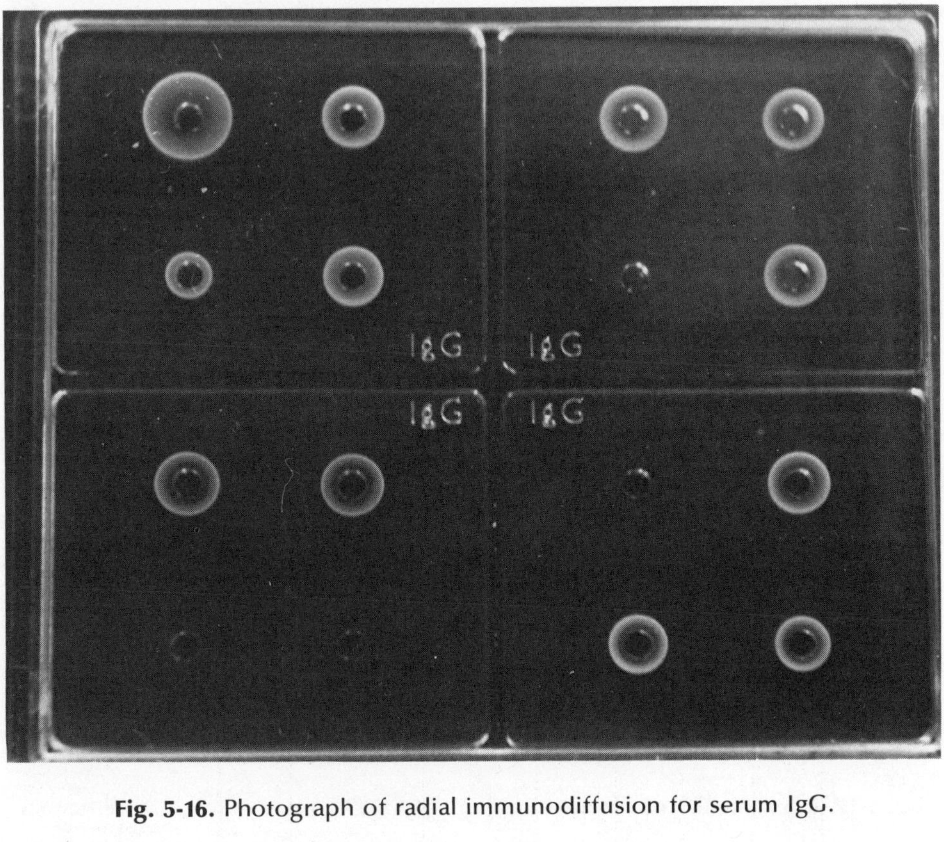

Fig. 5-16. Photograph of radial immunodiffusion for serum IgG.

ence technique for quantitation of serum proteins. In RID one of the two immune partners, usually antibody, is uniformly dispersed in a thin layer of agar or agarose. Small wells are cut into the agarose and a precise quantity of serum, standards, or controls is added (Fig. 5-16) to each well. If antibody is in the agarose, one would be detecting the specific antigen in the sera, controls, and standards. The agar plate is then incubated in a humid place, while the serum diffuses radially into the immunogel. As in Oudins' assay, precipitation occurs when the antigen-antibody ratio is at equivalence. As more serum diffuses, the precipitate solubilizes due to zonal phenomena, and the precipitate ring appears to migrate away from the well. When all antigen is consumed in antigen-antibody complexes, migration ceases. The size of this precipitin ring then is proportional to the antigen concentration in the sample.

A problem for the immunochemist has been to determine exactly what is the relationship between ring size and antigen concentration. It was found that the area of the precipitin ring best correlated to the ratio of antibody to antigen. Clearly the higher the antibody-to-antigen ratio the smaller the precipitin ring. Presently two variations in the general methodology are employed. In one, the limit or end point assay, the time of diffusion is such that ring growth is complete. This technique, developed by Mancini and Heremans, plots the square of the diameter of the standard rings versus concentration of these standards. The Mancini-Hereman assay results in a linear plot (Fig. 5-17, *A*). The second method, that of Fahey and McKelvey, is a timed assay. In this test samples, standards, and controls are allowed to diffuse for a precise time, approximately 18 hours or

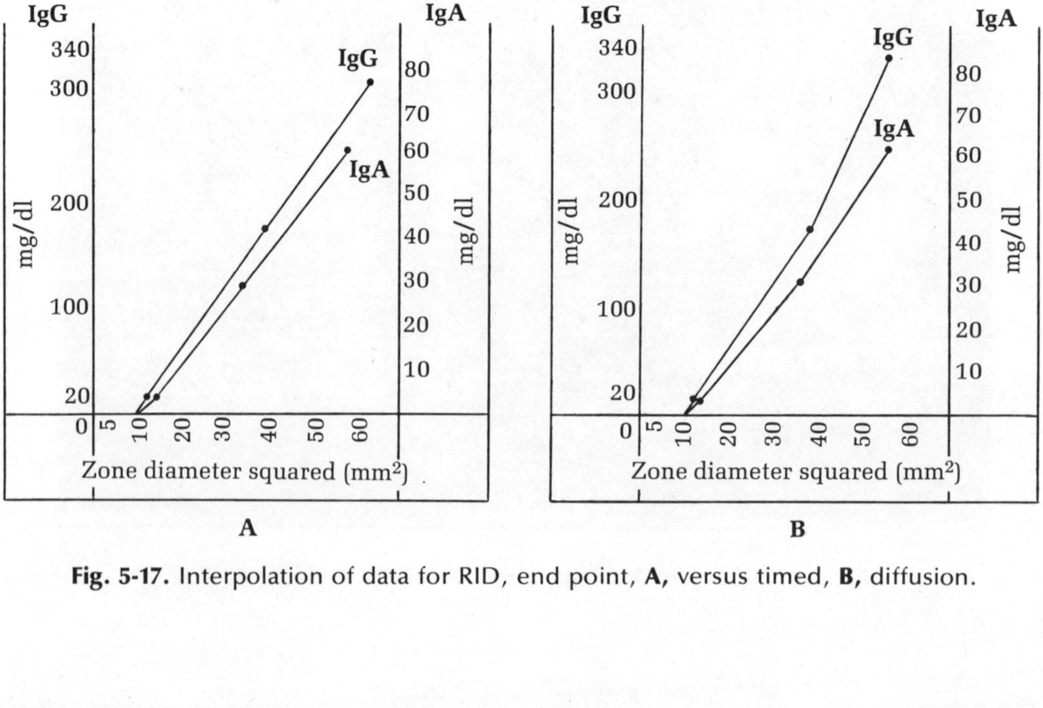

Fig. 5-17. Interpolation of data for RID, end point, **A,** versus timed, **B,** diffusion.

according to the manufacturers directions. In the timed assay, the plot is roughly linear when the log of the antigen concentration is plotted versus the diameter of the ring (note Fig. 5-17, *B*). Mancini's limit diffusion assay utilizes a higher percent antibody concentration in agar, hence it is able to immobilize the precipitate ring. The timed assay, with its lower antibody concentration, results in a continuously growing ring that may diffuse to the limits of the agar. Generally the Mancini method, because of its use of high antibody concentration, can be used as a timed or limit assay. It is thought that the timed assays are less reliable and that the end point diffusions are more precise at the expense of time. Some of the more common sources of errors include distortions or nicks in the agar, antigen or antibody excess, antigen spill, and the presence of polymeric antigen forms.

The simplicity of RID is of major importance but this is far outweighed by its specificity and sensitivity. The lowest detectable concentration of antigen in RID has been shown to be 1.25 μg/ml. With this sensitivity, RID becomes an assay with enormous potential. Kits presently available commercially include prealbumin, alpha$_1$-antitrypsin, transferrin, complement fraction C3, haptoglobin, immunoglobulins, light chains, and CRP among others.

Alpha$_1$-antitrypsin (AAT)

An inherited deficiency of alpha$_1$-antitrypsin (AAT) has clearly been shown to be related to emphysema. Detection of an AAT deficiency can provide the individual with an early and valuable warning. Substances and environments known to aggravate emphysema can be eliminated and may inhibit the progress of this malady. AAT is a protein that inhibits endoproteases, particularly trypsin. In the normal person inhalation of inflammatory debris results in a cellular response leading to phagocytosis and enzyme release. These proteolytic enzymes would be destined to autodestroy lung tissue if it were not for the serum enzyme inhibitor AAT. People with genetic deficiencies of this protein develop lung damage when exposed to respiratory inflammatory agents, such as in smoking. An important application of this assay is in employment counseling for hazardous occupations.

Methodology. Agar containing anti-AAT is layered onto a Petri dish. Wells are cut out of the agar with a template or capillary tubes. Three concentrations of reference standards are added to three wells. A control serum sample is added to the fourth well, and patient serum samples are added to the remaining wells. Using the timed assay system, the ring diameters are measured at 18 hours. The log of the antigen concentration for each standard is plotted versus that standard's ring diameter. This is easily accomplished via semilog graph paper (Fig. 5-17, *B*). The ring diameters of the control and patient's serum are measured and the antigen concentration is interpolated from the dose-response curve.

Interpretation. The normal person has an AAT of approximately 212 mg/dl serum. Heterozygous deficiencies result in AAT levels in the order of 125 mg/dl. The homozygous deficient person may have an AAT of 0 to 47 mg/dl. AAT may be increased in several disorders such as chronic pulmonary disease, gastric diseases, and liver diseases among others; AAT is normally increased in pregnancy.

Immunoglobulins

Excesses and deficiencies of immunoglobulins are associated with a variety of disorders. Accurate evaluation of immunoglobulin blood levels not only aids in confirming a diagnosis but also establishes the immune capability of the patient. RID is the reference method for assessment of immunoglobulin concentration in blood and certain other body fluids.

Methodology. Monospecific antiserum is prepared via animal immunization with pooled, purified immunoglobulins. The antiserum is absorbed with the various proteins in order to remove unwanted specificity. The resultant antibodies are primarily directed at the Fc region of each immunoglobulin. Once tested for specificity and potency, the antisera is incorporated into an agar layer. The general protocol described earlier is followed.

Interpretation. The normal values for serum immunoglobulins are discussed in Chapter 2. It should be emphasized that these values are age dependent. Recently growing interest in amniotic IgM has further expanded the value of this assay. The presence of an intrauterine fetal infection may be detected via elevated amniotic IgM. Low-level plates, commercially available, incorporate adjusted antibody concentration in agar and are ideal for measuring cerebrospinal fluid IgG. Spinal fluid IgG assays aid in the diagnosis of multiple sclerosis. A frequent source of error in RID estimation of immunoglobulins is the presence of polymeric forms in serum. For example, a normal individual may have 7S IgM, 19S IgM, or even 23S IgM while the standard for reference is 19S IgM. These various forms will diffuse into agar with different characteristics and may result in multiple rings and most likely misleading data. Another problem area is in the protein profile. If a patient has been shown to have an M component by protein electrophoresis, RID estimation of immunoglobulins is unreliable. Remember that monoclonal responses produce homogenous immunoglobulin such as pure IgG_2. However, the antisera are against all types of IgG and the standards are composed of all subclasses, hence one is comparing apples to oranges. Quantitation of M components is best made via protein electrophoresis.

Haptoglobin (Hp)

Haptoglobin (Hp) is a genetically controlled glycoprotein that demonstrates much polymorphism. It is composed of two alpha$_2$-globulin subunits. Three genetically distinct phenotypes exist, Hp 1-1, Hp 2-1, and Hp 2-2. Haptoglobulin functions to conserve body iron. Hp acts as a first line of defense in preservation of iron during intravascular hemolysis. Hemoglobin forms a stable complex with Hp and, as such, is unable to pass through the glomeruli. A decrease in free haptoglobin or a decrease in hemoglobin-binding capacity can be interpreted as an indication of hemolysis. Because of the heterogeneity of Hp, it is difficult to prepare an RID system that will contain standards comparable to that which each patient may demonstrate. Because of the heterogeneity of Hp, RID is not the most reliable technique to estimate Hp. When RID is used, the end point technique is preferred in order that migration of each form is complete.

Methodology. The technique is already described for RID. Each well is filled with serum samples, controls, or standards and is allowed to complete diffusion into monospecific immunogel. After cessation of ring migration, the squared diameters of the standards are plotted versus their Hp concentration. Values for patients and controls are interpolated from this dose-response curve.

Interpretation. The normal range is from 50 to 220 mg Hp/dl serum. Variations are encountered in several disorders as shown in the boxed material.

ELECTROIMMUNODIFFUSION (EID)

Serum protein

Commonly refered to as the Laurell "rocket", electroimmunodiffusion (EID) provides the clinical laboratory with a novel, fast, and accurate technique to estimate serum proteins. Until recently, the major limitation has been that the protein under study must have an electrophoretic mobility different than that of the antisera. EID combines immunochemical specificity with speed of electrophoresis.

Methodology. Plates are coated with immunogel. Patient samples, controls, and reference standards are applied to the immunogel and then electrophoresed across the plate. The pH of the buffered immunogel is such that the antiserum is at its pI, hence little movement occurs. As the samples rapidly migrate across the immunogel, narrow stationary precipitate bands form as the ratio of antigen and antibody approach equivalence. As shown in Fig. 5-18, the pattern of the precipitate band roughly resembles a rocket. The length of this rocket is proportional to antigen concentration.

Interpretation. Many of the same problems known to occur with radial diffusion also occur in EID. The presence of M components will again result in mis-

Free haptoglobin serum concentrations in various physiologic states

Decreased	Increased
Newborn	Pregnancy
Hemolytic anemia	Estrogen treatment
Transfusion reaction	Chronic infections
Hepatocellular disease	Inflammatory conditions
	Tissue destruction
	Obstructive jaundice

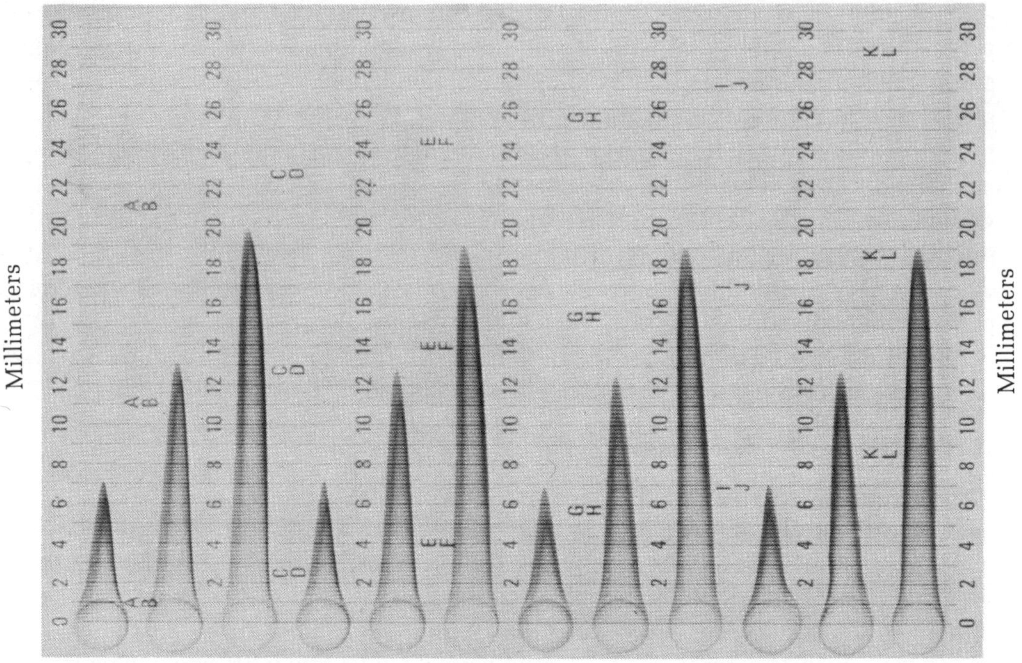

Fig. 5-18. Photograph of Laurell "rocket" electroimmunodiffusion. (Reprinted with permission of Millipore Corporation, Bedford, Massachusetts.)

leading data owing to problems discussed earlier. As with RID, EID may also be affected by zonal difficulties. The major advantage of EID is the time saved. EID kits are commercially available (Millipore Corporation, Bedford, Mass.) for alpha$_1$-antitrypsin, albumin, ceruloplasmin, alpha$_2$-globulin, transferrin, C3 fraction of complement and of course for IgG, IgA, and IgM.

Complement C3 fraction

The complement system will be discussed in detail in Chapter 7. Complement is a system of 11 separate protein components. These proteins are sequentially activated via the binding of IgG and IgM antibodies with antigens. An alternate pathway for activation of complement occurs through the binding of IgA, IgG_4, or IgE. In the alternate system the early complement components C1, C4, and C2 are bypassed and activation is initiated with C3. The component C3 is composed of an alpha chain, 110,000 daltons, and a beta chain, 70,000 daltons. This fraction is synthesized by the liver parenchymal cells and is important in the inflammatory process.

Methodology. C3 can be evaluated via the hemolytic capacity of complement or by immunochemical means. Recently, there has been increased interest in EID as an assay method for C3. Patient samples, controls, and reference standards are applied to a monospecific immunoagarose plate. The samples are elec-

Conditions accompanied by abnormal C3 levels

Decreased	Increased
Systemic lupus erythematosus	Necrotic disorders
Glomerulonephritis	
Immune complex disease	
Liver disease	

trophoresed for 2 hours, resulting in the formation of rocket-shaped precipitin bands. The length of these rockets is proportional to the concentration of C3.

Interpretation. Complement fraction C3 is frequently decreased in the serum of patients with markedly increased immune activity. It appears the mechanism for this decrease is not merely simple utilization of available C3. The adult normal is 96 to 150 mg C3/dl serum.

READINGS AND RESOURCES

Alpert, M. E., Uriel, J., and Nechaud, B.: Alpha-fetoprotein in the diagnosis of human hepatoma, N. Engl. J. Med. **278:**984-986, 1968.

Berne, B. H.: Differing methodology and equations used in quantitating immunoglobulins by radial immunodiffusion-A comparative evaluation of reported and commercial techniques, Clin. Chem. **20:**61-69, 1974.

Cowley, L. P.: Specific precipitation in gels and its application to immunological analysis, Methods Med. Res. **5:**335-378, 1942.

Fahey, J. L., and McKelvey, E. M.: Quantitative determination of serum immunoglobulins in antibody agar plates, J. Immunol. **94:**84-90, 1965.

Gitlin, D.: Normal biology of alpha-fetoprotein, Ann. N.Y. Acad. Sci. **259:**7-16, 1975.

Grant, G. H., and Butt, W. R.: Immunochemical methods in clinical chemistry, Adv. Clin. Chem. **13:**383-466, 1970.

Heidleberger, M., and Kendall, F. E.: A quantitative study of the precipitin reaction between type III pneumococcal polysaccharide and purified homologous antibody, J. Exp. Med. **50:**809-823, 1929.

Heremans, J. F., and Masson P. L.: Specific analysis of immunoglobulins. Techniques and clinical value, Clin. Chem. **19:**294-300, 1973.

Hutchison, D. C. S.: Alpha-antitrypsin deficiency and pulmonary emphysema. The role of protease enzymes and their inhibitors, Br. J. Dis. Chest. **67:**171, 1973.

Kohler, P. F., and Muller-Eberhard, H. J.: Immunochemical quantitation of the third, fourth and fifth components of the human complement: concentrations in the serum of healthy adults, J. Immunol. **99:**1211-1216, 1967.

Lourell, C. B.: Quantitative estimation of proteins by electrophoresis in agarose gel containing antibodies, Anal. Biochem. **15:**45-52, 1962.

Mancini, G., Corbonara, A. O., and Heremans, J. F.: Immunochemical quantitation of antigens by single radial diffusion, Immunochemistry **2:**237, 1965.

Miesch, F., Bieth, J., and Metais, P.: The alpha-I-antitrypsin and alpha-two-macroglobulin content and protease inhibiting capacity of normal and pathologic sera, Clin. Chim. Acta. **31:**231-241, 1971.

Oudin, J.: Specific precipitation in gels and its application to immunological analysis, Methods Med. Res. **5:**335-378, 1942.

Ritzman, S. E., and Daniels, J. C.: Serum protein abnormalities. Boston, 1975, Little, Brown & Co.

Roentree, R. J., and Rantz, L. A.: Clinical experience with the C-reactive protein test, Arch. Intern. Med. **96:**674-682, 1955.

Rose, N. R., and Bigazzi, P. E. editors: Methods

in immunodiagnosis, New York, 1973, John Wiley & Sons.

Rose, N. R. and Friedman, H., editors: Manual of clinical immunology, ASM Washington D.C., 1976.

Sleeper, C. A., and Cowley, L. P.: Detection of monoclonal gammopathy, Am. J. Clin. Pathol. **51:**395, 1965.

Tietz, N. W. editor: Fundamentals of clinical chemistry, Philadelphia, 1976, W. B. Saunders Co.

Williams, R. C. Jr., Bailey, R. C., and Howe, R. B.: Studies on benign serum M-components, Am. J. Med. Sci. **257:**277-293, 1969.

CHAPTER 6

Agglutination tests

Twenty years ago exotic laboratory glassware symbolized clinical laboratory medicine. Today the general public imagines the rapid glass slide assays as the symbol of laboratory work. Although these sensitive techniques are capable of performing only a fraction of the necessary tests, they do ease the overwhelming burden of modern medical technology. The fundamental principle of these assays is dependent on the reaction of particulate antigen with antibody. This reaction leads to a macroscopically visible agglutination. Agglutination tests are now used in endocrinology, toxicology, clinical chemistry, microbiology, and immunohematology among other disciplines of clinical laboratory medicine.

PRINCIPLES AND LIMITATIONS OF AGGLUTINATION TESTS

Agglutination is a secondary manifestation of the antibody-antigen reaction. The primary distinction between the precipitin assay and the agglutination assay is that in the precipitin assay antigen is soluble, no particles are present. In the basic agglutination test the antigen is particulate. Most of these particulate antigens range from 100 to 1000 times the size of antibody. For this reason relatively few antibody molecules are needed to elicit a visible clumping of the particles. Why agglutination occurs or how it occurs has been disputed. One theory states that because of surface charge, particles tend to repel each other. However, when the particle reacts with a sufficient number of antibody molecules, the charge changes allowing adherence of particles to each other. Most available research favors the lattice theory to explain the agglutination phenomena. As described earlier (precipitin, Chapter 5), the lattice theory holds that an immune complex grows in size. This growth continues because of the reaction of free antigenic determinants on the particle binding with Fab regions of the antibody molecule (Fig. 6-1). Antibody glues antigen particles together into a visible clump.

The agglutination reaction like the precipitin reaction occurs in two major steps, combination and aggregation. Combination is extremely rapid, while ag-

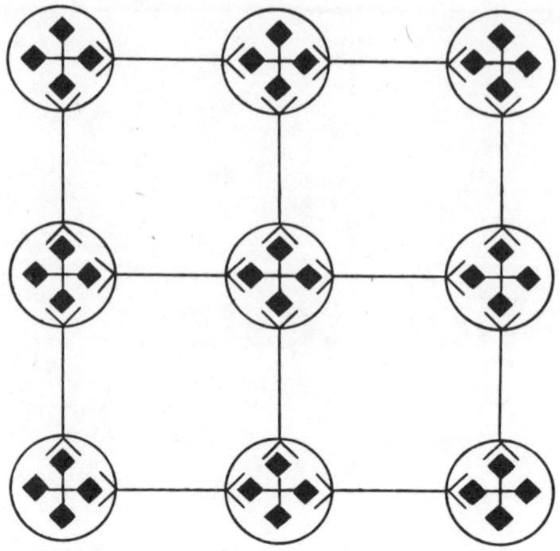

Fig. 6-1. Lattice theory in agglutination reactions. Particles with numerous antigenic determinants are bound together through reaction with antibodies.

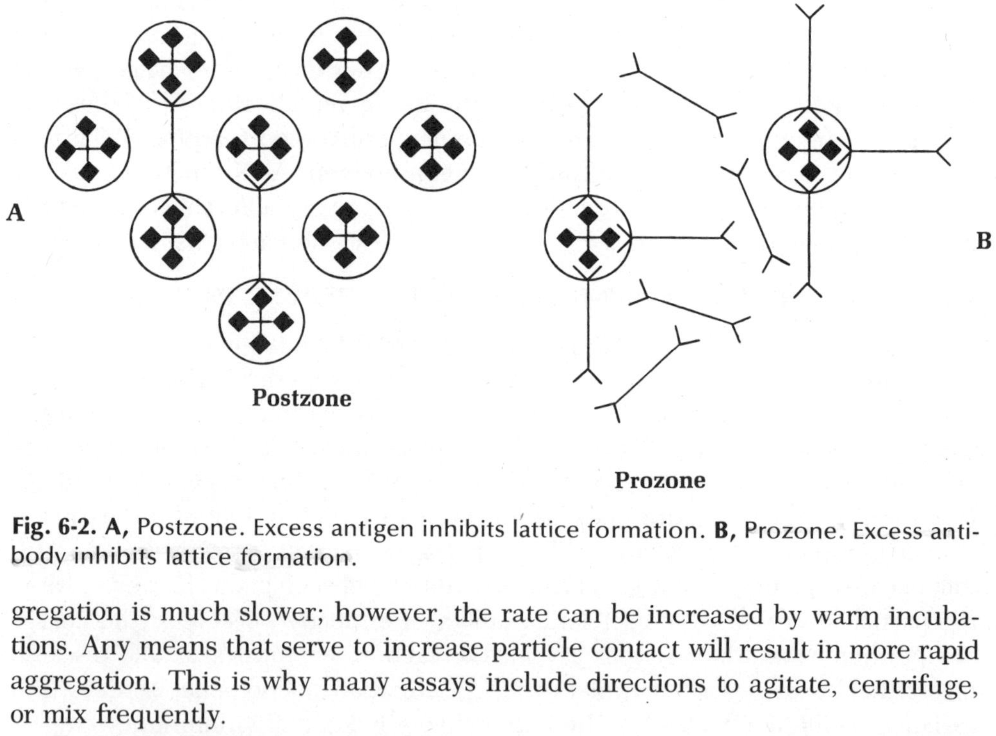

Fig. 6-2. A, Postzone. Excess antigen inhibits lattice formation. **B,** Prozone. Excess antibody inhibits lattice formation.

gregation is much slower; however, the rate can be increased by warm incubations. Any means that serve to increase particle contact will result in more rapid aggregation. This is why many assays include directions to agitate, centrifuge, or mix frequently.

Zonal phenomena occur often in agglutination assays. As shown in Fig. 6-2, excess antigen or antibody can inhibit lattice formation and may cause a negative reaction. Most agglutination reaction assays use an initial serum dilution to counter the effects of excess antibody. Because particles settle rapidly, improper mixing may enhance zonal problems.

Surface charges on particles can frequently cause problems in reading agglutination reactions. In general, inert particles tend to aggregate in solution but cellular particles, particularly red blood cells, have the opposite problem. When red blood cells are suspended in aqueous media with low ionic strengths, there is a tendency to develop a negative cloud of ions around each cell. This cloud of negative charges causes repulsion between cells, inhibiting agglutination. For this reason all agglutination reactions are performed in an electrolyte medium. The electrolyte, such as 0.15 M NaCl, dampens the net negative charge. With charges neutralized, cells can approach each other to allow separate Fab fragments of single antibody molecules to bridge the space between cells. Often other buffers such as Veronal-buffered saline solution or glycine-buffered saline solution are used for this same purpose; albumins, polyvinylprolidione, and dextrans are also used.

Positive and negative controls are critical to agglutination tests. The value of the positive control is somewhat obvious, and most people require little persuasion to incorporate its use with routine assaying of patient samples. Simply stated the use of the positive control verifies the antigenic activity of the particles and reminds the analyst what a positive reaction should look like. Many more subtle errors in procedures and preparation of reagents may be recognized by the failure of the positive control to react in a typical fashion. These subtle errors may include improper mixing of reagents and contamination of reagents, glassware, and/or patient samples. The negative control ensures the fact that the antigen particles are not oversensitive and that they remain smooth and finely granular in the absence of reacting antibody. The negative control also aids the analyst in reading trace reactions by clearly observing a real negative reaction with each assay.

It was thought for many years that certain antibodies were precipitins and that others were agglutinins. It was shown that the agglutinins were IgM antibodies. We know today that this is not always true. Many reaction specificities are determined by the type of antigen. For example, polysaccharide antigens, as found in the bacterial cell, normally elicit a strong IgM response. Since IgM has a high avidity, large size, and multiple Fab fragments, IgM antibody reacts well in agglutinating systems. On the other hand, soluble protein antigens tend to elicit strong IgG reactions and therefore react well in precipitin tests. Many current modifications of the basic agglutination test have proved that some IgG's can be agglutinins although not as effectively as the IgM class of antibodies.

Methodology. The basic procedure for agglutination test titration involves:

1. Serial dilution of patient serum (twofold or tenfold)
2. Addition of equivalent volumes of antigen suspension
3. Incubation at 37° C with agitation
4. Visual observation of macroscopic agglutination

The end point is considered to be that dilution in which 50% of the antigen is agglutinated. For convenience and simplicity, since it may be difficult to observe this 50% point, many laboratories report the titer (serum potency) as the last dilution that shows visible agglutination; consistency is of primary importance. The titer is reported as the reciprocal of the dilution.

Today there are several popular techniques or modifications of the basic agglutination procedure. The first, the macrotube technique, uses large amounts of patient sample and reagents and is performed in test tubes. Many microtechniques are gaining in popularity. These techniques use special equipment to reduce time-reagent volume and patient sample. Another adaptation of the agglutinin assay is the slide test. Using droppers and marked glass slides, reagents are added and mixed and macroscopic agglutination is observed (Fig. 6-3). Most slide tests emphasize the importance of reading at a precise time, for example, "rock slide gently and observe for agglutination in two minutes." The reason for this emphasis is that small quantities are used over a fairly large area; therefore one may be easily misled by the effects of evaporation. The slide test is often used as a qualitative screening test to determine if the patient has a particular antibody. By serially diluting serum sample and then testing a drop of each dilution it is possible to roughly estimate titer. The tube assay is generally considered to be the most reliable technique; however, excellent results are obtained by the experienced technologist using microtitration systems.

Agglutination reactions are very sensitive; the antigen particle is large in

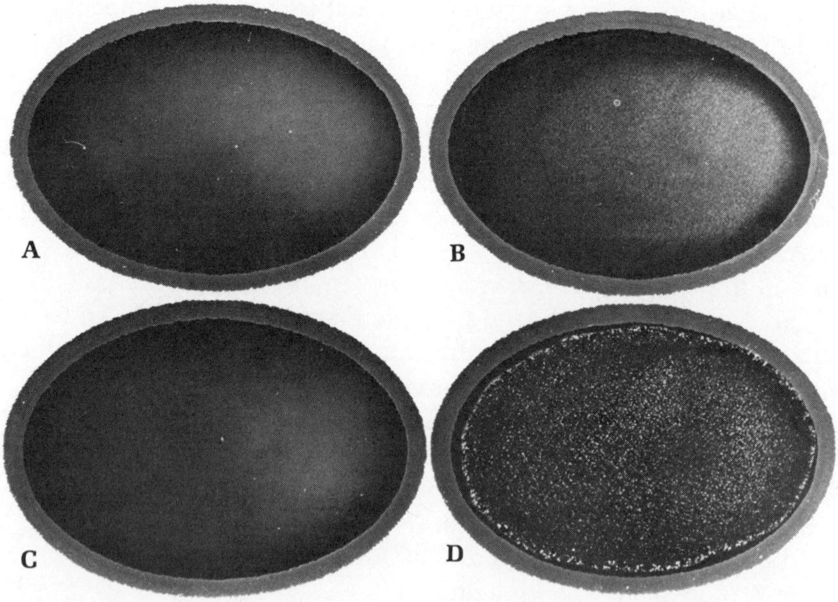

Fig. 6-3. Macroscopic slide agglutination test for rheumatoid factor. Note **A,** negative agglutination; **B,** rough agglutination, or weakly reactive; **C,** negative agglutination; and **D,** positive agglutination. (Courtesy of Hyland, Costa Mesa, California.)

comparison to antibody. Therefore relatively few antibody molecules are needed to demonstrate a positive test. Although agglutination tests are very sensitive, they are not very precise. In estimating the 50% agglutination end point, a single tube error in a twofold dilution system yields ± 100% variation. For these very reasons the agglutination phenomenon is most suitable for qualitative testing.

DIRECT AGGLUTINATION TESTS

The most basic agglutination procedure is the direct test. Direct agglutination tests can be used to detect specific antibodies with known antigens or conversely specific antigens with known antibodies. For example, a bacterial suspension may be used to identify antibodies in infectious diseases, or anti-A and anti-B may be used to identify the patients' blood group antigens. One must be aware of the fact that particulate antigens, for example, bacteria and cells, contain a wide variety of diverse antigens, some of which may appear on other nonrelated particles. This diversity may lead to cross-reactions, interference, or even blocking of antigenic sites.

Widal test

A definitive diagnosis of bacterial, mycotic, rickettsial, and viral infections is best accomplished through the culture, isolation, and identification of the offending organism. However, isolation is frequently a difficult or impossible task. Detecting antibodies to the organism may further support a diagnosis. There are many problems encountered in attempting this type of indirect diagnosis. One must consider the patient's history, for recent or past infections or immunizations may result in persistent titers not related to the present illness. In many areas of the country people develop natural antibodies because of the prevalence of particular antigens. Cross-reactive antibodies and heterologous antigens may complicate the diagnostic picture. Occasionally, a patient may have an immune deficiency, which is in reality the cause of the infection making the patient incapable of developing a humoral antibody response. The immune-deficient patient may indeed have no detectable antibody to a particular organism, while in fact exhibiting the infectious disease symptoms because of that agent.

Some bacteria exhibit two broad clinically useful types of antigens, "H" and "O." The "H" antigens are those related to the flagella of motile organisms. When antibody reacts with these antigens in vitro, a flocculent reaction occurs, presumably owing to the tangling of the flagella. The flocculant is soft and puffy in character while still fitting into the definition of agglutination. This type of agglutination is easily dispersed by agitation. Reaction of antibody with "O" type antigens (somatic) produces a rough granular agglutinate, which resists dispersion by agitation.

Principles. The Widal test is an agglutination immunoassay used to aid in the diagnosis of *Salmonella* infections. Approximately 98% of the pathogenic *Salmonella* in the United States belong to five major serologic groups—A, B, C,

D, and E. The "O" antigens of these organisms are remarkably stable between groups, while the "H" antigen displays much variation. Cultured isolates may contain combinations of species- and group-specific flagellar antigens. Any culture that exhibits only species-specific antigens is considered monophasic; cultures that exhibit both are diphasic.

A third group of antigens (bacterial envelope) are also helpful in diagnosing patients with *Salmonella typhi* infections. Antibodies to these antigens rapidly disappear from the serum after the active infection. Hence, detection of the antibodies to these antigens is highly suggestive of current infection. The abbreviation "Vi" is used to describe these antigens. Patients exhibiting "Vi" antibodies may be carriers responsible for epidemic spread of the infectious disease. Although the Widal test is accomplished most frequently via a slide dilution method, the macrotube test is considered, and has proved to be, more accurate and more reliable.

Methodology. As described in the basic protocol, tubes are labeled and an initial 1:10 dilution of patient serum is twofold diluted serially with saline solution. A separate row of ten tubes is used for each antigen to be tested. The last tube of each row is used as a negative control and therefore should contain only saline solution. Well-mixed equal volumes of bacterial antigens are added to each tube, including the control. During the incubation time the tubes are periodically mixed by shaking the rack. At the end of the incubation the tubes are inspected for agglutination, which appears as clumps of organisms when mildly agitated.

Periodic testing with a known positive control serum is necessary to ensure the standardization of the antigen suspension and the reactivity of the antigenic determinants.

Interpretation. The last tube showing macroscopically visible agglutination is considered the end point, and the reciprocal of that dilution is the titer. Because of the high frequency of prozone reaction in bacterial infection, it is imperative to test all dilutions. Interpretation of the titer of each assay is very difficult. There are a great many variables, discussed earlier, that affect the titer for each patient. Changes in titer in the acute and convalescent specimens are more readily inter-

Table 13. Weil-Felix reactions in rickettsial diseases

Disease	Proteus antigens		
	OX-19	OX-2	OX-K
Epidemic typhus	++++	+	0
Murine endemic typhus	++++	+	0
Scrub typhus (tsutsugamushi)	0	0	+++
Rocky Mountain spotted fever	++++	+	0
Rickettsialpox	0	0	0
Q fever	0	0	0

preted. Antibodies to flagellate antigens appear later in the course of the illness and the titer reaches a late peak. The "O" titer drops off rapidly during the convalescent stage. A titer of 1 : 160 or above for "H" and "O" antigens, in the unvaccinated individual, is highly suggestive of infection.

Weil-Felix reactions (WF)

In 1916, Weil and Felix isolated a strain of *Proteus* from a patient with typhus. Suprisingly this organism was agglutinated by the serum of other patients with typhus fever. The original *Proteus* strain used in this test was OX-19. However, strains OX-2 and OX-K were also found useful for the diagnosis of other rickettsial diseases. The mechanism for this reactivity is not completely understood. This cross-reactivity may be due to polyfunctional binding of antibody to a common antigenic determinant. Both *Rickettsia prowazekii* and *Proteus* OX-19 display a common polysaccharide that may be the source of this cross-reactivity.

Interpretation. Although not a specific test, the WF is useful in diagnosing rickettsial diseases. WF antibodies appear early, 6 to 12 days after infection. The titer reaches a peak during early convalescence, and the antibody is usually undetectable 5 months after clinical recovery.

Brucella and tularemia

Brucellosis in humans is clinically similar to many other disorders. Detection of antibodies is useful in aiding diagnosis, and absence of brucella antibodies helps rule out this organism as the causative agent. Three antigenically related organisms are responsible for this disorder: *Brucella abortus*, *Brucella melitensis*, and *Brucella suis*. For this reason an antigen preparation from any one of the three organisms is suitable to detect antibodies to any of the three organisms. Although titers persist for many years after infection, a titer of 320 in the presence of symptoms is considered definitive.

Francisella tularensis is the causative agent for tularemia. The organisms is extremely difficult to isolate and culture. A diagnosis of tularemia is often based on the result of this agglutination test. Rising titers are the most indicative finding for tularemia, while undetectable antibody does not rule out this disease.

Cold agglutinins

Principles. Antibodies reactive in the cold with adult human red blood cells are found in the serum of 34% to 68% of the patients with *Mycoplasma pneumoniae* infections. The antibody appears to react with erythrocyte stromata receptors. The ideal would be to isolate and identify the causative agent of this atypical pneumonia. However, culture and isolation of the mycoplasma organism is extremely difficult and unreliable. Direct hemagglutination of human red blood cells offers the clinical laboratory a means to aid in the diagnosis. The "thermal amplitude" (the reactive temperature range) is between 0° and 20° C and the bonding is reversible. At cold temperatures a positive serum will agglutinate group O human red blood cells and when warmed to body temperature the agglutinated red blood cells will dissociate.

Methodology. Twofold serial dilutions of the patient's serum with saline solution are tested with group O human red blood cells. Group O cells are used to avoid the influence of the patient's naturally occurring anti-A or anti-B. The cell-serum dilutions are incubated for 1 hour at 4° C and immediately are inspected for agglutination. If the reaction seen is due to cold agglutinins, clumped cells will disperse when warmed to 37° C.

Interpretation. There is limited value to single titers; more information is obtained from sequential testing. The most frequently encountered source of error stems from a lack of understanding of the behavior of the cold agglutinin. If the patient's blood sample (cells and serum) is stored in a refrigerator, the cold agglutinins will be removed from the serum and will coat the cells, resulting in a false negatively reacting serum. This common error can be easily overcome by preincubation of patient's blood at 37° C prior to centrifugation before testing.

Infectious mononucleosis

Infectious mononucleosis (IM) is an acute self-limiting infectious disease caused by the Epstein-Barr virus. It is most frequently seen in young adults and adolescents who display a characteristic clinical picture of pharyngitis and lymphadenopathy with a marked increase in peripheral atypical lymphocytes. The signs and symptoms of IM are rather nonspecific, and the clinical picture may remarkably resemble more severe conditions such as lymphocytic leukemia. During 1935 to 1937, Davidsohn developed a differential agglutinin test that was a major improvement over earlier presumptive tests.

Davidsohn differential

Principles. Heterophil antibodies are antibodies that react with phylogenetically unrelated antigens. Several conditions result in the production of anti-sheep agglutinins in man. Injection of Forssman antigens such as guinea pig, spleen, brain, adrenal, and kidney tissues into a rabbit induces the production of high titers of antibody to sheep red blood cells. Serum sickness, immunization with Forssman antigen, and IM virus all cause the production of heterophil antibody to sheep red blood cells. Earlier presumptive assays merely titered this sheep agglutinin without any effort to distinguish the cause. Davidsohn realized that boiled guinea pig kidney would absorb heterophil antibody produced by Forssman antigen or serum sickness, leaving the heterophil antibody owing to IM in the serum. He further employed beef red blood cells to specifically absorb antibodies caused by IM (Table 14).

Methodology. The Davidsohn heterophil test attempts to distinguish the causes of anti-sheep red blood cell titers. In the tube test, two rows of test tubes are labeled, one guinea pig, the other beef red blood cells. Inactivated serum is added to the first tube in each row and the appropriate antigen is added to each aliquot. The test is incubated at room temperature in order for absorption to oc-

Table 14. Differential Davidsohn heterophil for infectious mononucleosis

Absorbing antigen	Heterophil Ab absorbed	Titer to red blood cells		
		IM	SS	FA
Forssman (guinea pig) Ag	Forssman serum sickness	↑	↓	↓
Beef red blood cells	IM SS	↓	↓	↑

NOTE: SS = Serum sickness; FA = Forssman antigen; IM = Infectious mononucleosis.

cur. After centrifugation the absorbed sera are titered with sheep red blood cells and saline solution.

Interpretation. Differential assay is interpreted as shown in Table 14. The differential test is specific and qualitative. The actual titer of anti-sheep red blood cells is of little significance and no correlation exists between the titer and the severity of the disease. Recent efforts to reduce assay time have led to the proliferation of rapid slide tests.

Spot test for infectious mononucleosis. Lee, in 1968, relied on several basic observations and developed the first rapid differential IM assay. In his studies he found that horse red blood cells are more sensitive than sheep red blood cells to heterophil antibody. Horse red blood cells were found remarkably more stable than sheep red blood cells. Finally, he noted that guinea pig kidney and beef red blood cell stroma were capable of instant heterophil absorption (high affinity).

Methodology. Two areas of a glass slide are marked to isolate reagents. To one area patient serum and guinea pig antigen are added; to the other area patient serum and beef stroma are added. Both sets of serum and reagent are mixed thoroughly with clean wood applicator sticks prior to the addition of horse red blood cells. Horse erythrocytes are added to both areas and are observed for agglutination at precise times.

Interpretation. The results are interpreted according to Table 14. The test is considered highly specific and more sensitive than the differential tube test. Common sources of error include improper mixing of reagents, rouleau formation of cells, and unclean glassware. The spot test with horse red blood cells will detect IM earlier than nonhorse cell assays.

INDIRECT (PASSIVE) AGGLUTINATION

Certain substances will naturally adhere to surfaces of various particles. Once bound to the particle the soluble substance is capable of reacting with antibody. In this way it is possible to employ soluble antigens in agglutination reactions (Fig. 6-4). For example, soluble polysaccharides adhere to the surface of red blood cells. If one wishes to detect antibodies to the pneumococcal polysaccharide, it is relatively simple to use the passive hemagglutination assay. Red blood cells are mixed with purified pneumococcal polysaccharide and the excess

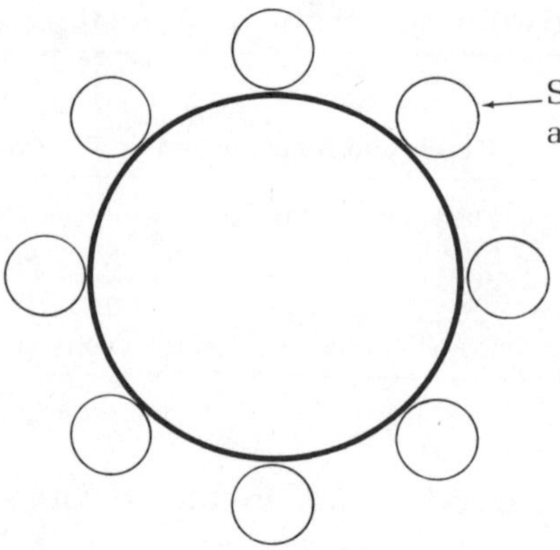

Fig. 6-4. Passive agglutination. Carrier particles (red blood cells, latex particles, and so on) coated with soluble antigen allow agglutination reactions to be used to detect antibodies to soluble antigens.

polysaccharide, not absorbed, is washed away. The red blood cells act as carriers of the antigen. The serum to be tested is serially diluted with saline solution and mixed with equal volumes of the red blood cell suspension. Again, as in the direct assay, one inspects the tube dilutions for hemagglutination. Special pretreatment of red blood cells is necessary in order to attach protein antigens to their surface. The most popular procedure called tannning utilizes tannic acid for treatment of red blood cells. Tannic acid appears to uncover protein receptors on the red cell surface. The process of tanning has several drawbacks, including weak binding of antigens to the red blood cell surface, and the increased fragility of cells frequently leads to hemolysis. Some assays use chromic acid–treated cells, which results in stronger interaction of antigen with red blood cells. Although cells are often used in passive agglutination tests, there are many other inert carrier particles such as latex and bentonite. Passive agglutination assays greatly expand the usefulness of agglutination tests and are extremely sensitive.

Rheumatoid factor

Rheumatoid factors (RF) are immunoglobulins directed at the Fc region of IgG molecules. Although RF is found in each class of immunoglobulins, most test systems are more sensitive to the IgM anti-IgG (Fc) type. Most RF analytical systems make use of human IgG bound to a variety of inert particles. The RF is readily detected via passive agglutination (Figs. 6-3 and 6-5).

Methodology. The most common technique is that of Singer and Plotz. In this assay human fraction II (IgG) is absorbed onto a suspension of latex particles. The assay is primarily a slide test. Serum is heat inactivated for 30 minutes at 56° C. This procedure is necessary to inactivate complement that may result in error with certain patients. A glass slide with well-marked oval areas is used to contain the reagents. One drop of 1 : 20 dilution of patient serum, positive control, and negative control is added to the appropriate areas. One drop of well-

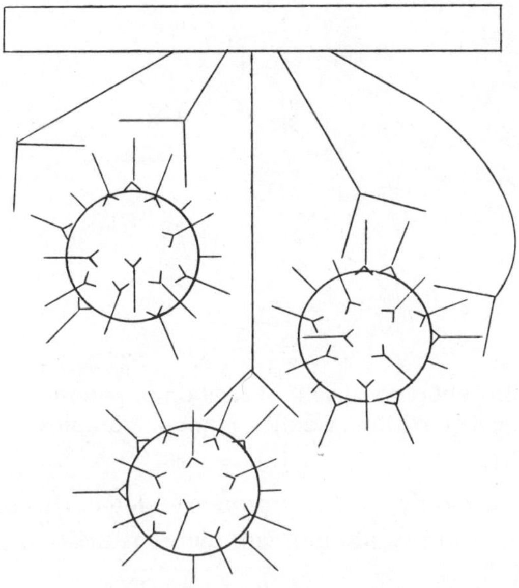

Fig. 6-5. Rheumatoid arthritis latex agglutination reaction. Patient's serum IgM anti-IgG reacts with IgG-coated latex particles.

mixed latex-antigen particles is added to each area and mixed thoroughly with wooden applicator sticks. The slide is rocked gently and inspected for macroscopic agglutination (Fig. 6-4).

Interpretation. High titers of RF are suggestive of rheumatoid arthritis, while titers of 20 or 80 are more difficult to evaluate. RF is often detected in the elderly and in patients with a variety of disorders. The disorders associated with positive rheumatoid factor include:

1. Acute immune responses (infectious mononucleosis)
2. Sarcoidosis
3. Systemic lupus erythematosus
4. Sjögrens syndrome

Several factors are responsible for infrequently encountered false positive tests, such as incomplete inactivation of complement, hyperlipidemia, and the presence of cryoglobulins. Certain patients may exhibit high titers of IgG-RF. These IgG-RF's will not be detected in most assays. Since IgG is bivalent and it contains the antigen, the Fc area, it is capable of self-reacting (Fig. 6-6). These intermediate complexes inhibit lattice formation but may appear in gel diffusion systems or in protein electrophoresis.

Antithyroid antibodies

Autoantibodies directed at thyroglobulins are associated with Hashimoto's thyroiditis. It is not clear whether the antibody is the cause of the thyroid abnormality or if it is the result of thyroid damage, for example, viral or surgical tissue

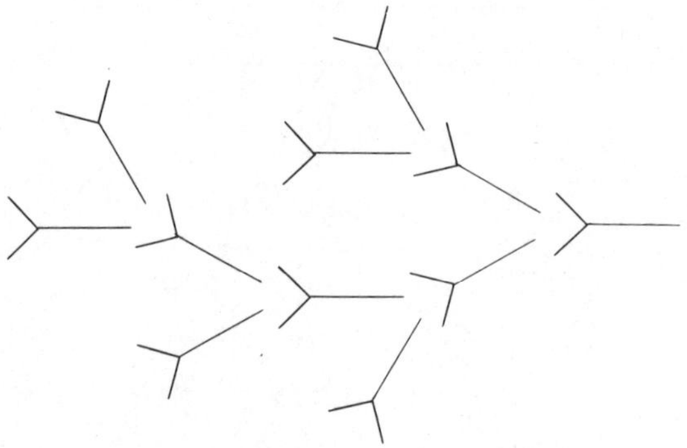

Fig. 6-6. Schematic representation of self-association of patient's serum IgG antibodies directed at their own IgG-Fc regions yielding immune complexes.

damage. The more commonly used techniques to detect this antibody are tanned red blood cell agglutination inhibition, complement fixation assays, and a latex (passive) agglutination.

Antinuclear factor (ANF)

Patients with systemic lupus erythematosus (SLE) develop a wide variety of immunologic abnormalities, including overresponsive B cells, deficiency of T cell function, and production of an array of autoantibodies. Antinuclear factor (ANF) is an IgG, 7S antibody directed at DNA and its associated proteins. It appears that the ANF is responsible for the classical LE phenomenon. Traumatized polynuclear cells are affected by antinuclear antibodies leading to phagocytosis of this swollen nuclear body. The classical LE preparation is laborious, somewhat unreliable, and insensitive.

Recently scientists have searched for more rapid, sensitive, and specific techniques. Today, with radioimmunoassay, it is now possible to accurately detect and quantitate anti-DNA (Farr technique). However a more rapid screening method is still of value. Commercially available passive latex kits for ANF are available. In these kits latex particles are coated with deoxyribonucleoprotein. The coated particles are tested with patient serum and positive and negative controls on glass slides. After thorough mixing, the suspensions are inspected for macroscopic agglutination. Although these tests are generally not considered more specific nor more sensitive than the LE preparation, they are less susceptible to error and are extremely fast. Anti-DNP titers are detected in 15% of the patients with rhematoid arthritis. A further discussion on antinuclear antibodies is included in Chapter 9.

PASSIVE AGGLUTINATION INHIBITION

The most sensitive modification of the basic agglutination test has promoted the use of this technique in the analysis of more esoteric substances. Agglutination inhibition assays utilize two reagents, inert antigen/hapten–coated particles and specific homologous antisera. Mixture of the two reagents produces agglutination. The basic principle of this assay is simply that if homologous antigen/hapten is present in the patient sample it can neutralize the antisera and inhibit agglutination. In this assay agglutination indicates the absence of antigen in the patient sample, while no agglutination indicates the presence of homologous antigen in the patient sample. Since no agglutination is a positive reaction, it is most important to include a positive and negative control with each assay. One should also consider that the antigen-particle suspension must be matched for each kit lot to reduce the possibility of zonal inhibition. Therefore one should discard leftover reagents rather than add them to new kits.

Human chorionic gonadotropin

Principles. Pituitary gonadotropins such as luteinizing hormone and thyroid-stimulating hormone are structurally related to human chorionic gonadotropin (HCG). HCG is a 40,000-dalton glycoprotein produced by the placenta. Since this hormone is produced by the placenta, its presence in patient serum or urine is indicative of pregnancy. The detection of HCG provides the clinical laboratory with a highly sensitive and specific pregnancy test. It is possible, via radioimmunoassay, to detect HCG a mere 8 days after conception. While it is possible to measure HCG by bioassay, agglutination inhibition (AI) offers the most rapid, economical, and expedient technique. The AI assays for HCG are 75% to 95% reliable for the normal pregnancy at 6 weeks past the first day of the last menstrual period.

Methodology. The patient urine sample is thoroughly mixed with anti-HCG. Presence of HCG in the patient's urine results in neutralization of antisera. After this step, HCG-coated latex is added and mixed well. If antisera were neutralized by patient HCG, then the antisera would fail to agglutinate the coated particles. On the other hand, if the person is not pregnant, then there is no HCG in the urine sample. The antisera remain reactive and agglutination results. A simple procedure is used for a tube assay.

Interpretation. The sensitivity of AI assays for HCG is approximately 1 to 2 international units. The test is extremely sensitive and reliable in normal pregnancy. Since HCG levels are outside of the normal limits in abnormal pregnancies, there has been some effort to use HCG titrations to monitor high-risk pregnancies. Specimens obtained from individuals with HCG-secreting tumors and moles will yield a positive test for pregnancy, for example, choriocarcinoma, hydatidiform mole, and testicular tumors. Some drugs have been shown to interfere with most immunologic pregnancy tests. Urine samples with low specific gravities and/or large amounts of drugs or bacteria may yield unreliable results.

Morphine

Principles. Immunochemistry has recently expanded its role in clinical toxicology. Increased needs to monitor therapeutic and abused drugs in body fluids have demanded more accurate, sensitive, and rapid analytical systems. Morphine

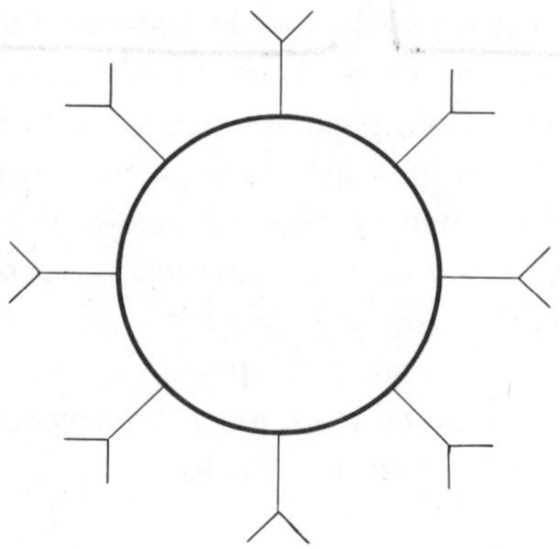

Fig. 6-7. Reverse indirect (passive) agglutination reaction utilizes particles coated with antibody to detect soluble antigen.

is the metabolic product of heroin. Morphine analysis has been adapted to hemagglutination-inhibition assay. This system is capable of detecting as little as 0.01 μg/ml of urine. Antisera are prepared via morphine-macromolecule complex immunization of experimental animals. The morphine is a hapten and with its carrier molecule induces antibody formation. The second reagent utilizes morphine bound to red blood cells. The presence of morphine in the patient sample effectively inhibits agglutination of the red blood cell–morphine complex.

Methodology. The patient sample is mixed with a precise amount of antibody to morphine. Two dilutions of patient sample are used to gain quantitative data. After 10 minutes of incubation sensitized red blood cells are added. The cells settle to the bottom of the tube in characteristic agglutination patterns.

Interpretation. The assay is so sensitive that it is impossible for the drug user to dilute out the urine concentration via excess imbibition of water. It is suggested that all positive hemagglutination assays be repeated by the more precise and conventional technique, gas/liquid chromatography. Several drugs with similar molecular structure interfere with the morphine immunoassay.

REVERSE PASSIVE AGGLUTINATION (RPA)

In the reverse passive agglutination (RPA) assays the Fc portion of antibody is bound to the inert carrier particles. This modification makes it possible to detect soluble antigens in the patient sample via agglutination tests (note Fig. 6-7).

C-reactive protein

Principles. As discussed previously, CRP is an acute phase reactive protein. An RPA assay for CRP is commercially available (Hyland, Costa Mesa, California). In these kits, latex particles are complexed with antibody to CRP. When these particles are mixed with CRP-positive serum, agglutination results.

Methodology. Inactivated serum, diluted 1:5 and 1:50 with glycine-buffered saline solution, is placed on separate areas of a glass slide. Negative and positive controls are pipetted to other labeled areas. One drop of anti-CRP particles is added to each area and thoroughly mixed. After 4 minutes of gentle rocking, the slide is examined for macroscopic agglutination.

Interpretation. The controls must display the appropriate reaction for the test to be considered accurate. Patient samples with titers greater than 50 should be further diluted to obtain the end point. The high frequency of elevated CRP makes it imperative to incorporate a 1:50 dilution in order to prevent false negative (postzone). Because the latex particles are coated with immunoglobulins in RPA assays, these particles will be reactive in the presence of RF. The results of latex CRP have been shown to correlate with precipitin CRP in 95.6% of the assays.

READINGS AND RESOURCES

Ager, J. A., Hutt, M. S. R., and Smith, G.: Detection of thyroid antibodies using bentonite particles, Nature **169:**307, 1959.

Allen, J. C., and Kunkel, A. G.: Hidden rheumatoid factors with specificity for native gamma globulin, Arthritis Rheum. **9:**758, 1966.

Boyden, S.: The absorption of proteins on erythrocytes treated with tannic acid and subsequent hemagglutination by anti-protein sera, J. Exp. Med. **93:**107, 1951.

Butler, W. T.: Hemagglutination studies with formalinized erythrocytes. Effect of bis-diazobenzidine and tannic acid treatment on sensitization by soluble antigens, J. Immunol. **90:** 663, 1963.

Davidsohn, I.: Heterophile antigens and antibodies, Arch. Pathol. **4:**776-801, 1927.

Davidsohn, I., and Henry, J. B.: Todd-Sanford clinical diagnosis by laboratory methods, ed. 15. Philadelphia, 1974, W. B. Saunders Co., pp. 1223-1224.

Dowdle, W. R., and Robinson, R. Q.: An indirect hemagglutination test for the diagnosis of *Mycoplasma pneumoniae* infections, Proc. Soc. Exp. Biol. Med. **116:**947, 1964.

Finegold, S. M., Martin, W. J., and Scott, E. G.: Bailey and Scott's diagnostic microbiology: a textbook for the isolation and identification of pathogenic microorganisms, ed. 5, St. Louis, 1978, The C. V. Mosby Co.

Garrow, D. H.: A rapid test for the presence of increased cold agglutinins, Br. Med. J. **11:**20, 1958.

Horowitz, C. A., Jerome, E., Diamond, R. and Ward, P. C. J.: Evaluation of latex tube agglutination-inhibition pregnancy test, Am. J. Obstet. Gynecol. **116:**626-632, 1973.

Rose, N. R., and Friedman, H., editor: Manual of clinical immunology, A.S.M. Washington, D.C., 1976.

Schroeder, S. A.: Interpretation of serologic tests for typhoid fever, J.A.M.A. **206:**839-840, 1968.

Shubert J. H., Holdman, L., and Moutin, D.S.: Evaluation of certain factors which effect the titers obtained in the Weil-Felix test, J. Lab. Clin. Med. **44:**194, 1954.

Singer, J. M., and Plotz, C. M.: The latex fixation test I, Am. J. Med. **21:**888, 1956.

Tillet, W. B., and Francis, T. O.: Serological reaction in pneumonia with a non-protein somatic fraction of pneumococcus, J. Exp. Med. **52:**561, 1930.

Welch, H., and Mickle, F. L.: A rapid slide test for serological diagnosis of typhoid and paratyphoid fevers, Am. J. Public Health. **26:**248, 1936.

Weil, E., and Felix, A.: Zur serogischem diagnose des fleckfiebers, Wien. Klin. Wochenschr. **29:**2, 1916.

CHAPTER 7

Complement

Pfeiffer, in 1894, noted that certain bacteria when injected into the intraperitoneal cavity of guinea pigs immediately disintegrated. To his surprise this phenomenon was reproducible in vitro. If the guinea pig serum was preincubated at 56° C for 30 minutes, this bacterial lytic activity was lost. When the preincubated serum-bacterial suspension was "spiked" with normal nonimmune serum, lytic activity was restored. Just what did all this mean? Early researchers concluded that normal serum contained a third factor. This factor called "alexin" (Greek, to ward off) was heat labile and was responsible for lytic activity. Today we know the third factor to be complement, a system of proteins that "complements" the action of antigen and antibody. Many of the activities often attributed to the antigen-antibody reaction are in reality due to complement. Complement plays a major role in the defense of the body, and unfortunately, often plays a role in inflicting damage to one's own tissues. Complement also is utilized in a sensitive and precise immune assay system. This chapter includes the nomenclature used in the complement system and details the mechanisms of activation. It is important to understand the role of complement in normal immune defense and in immunopathology. One should be aware of the intricacies, uses, and limitations, of the complement fixation test.

COMPLEMENT SYSTEM

Nomenclature

Complement is actually a system of 11 distinct proteins that make up about 10% of the total globulin fraction. These proteins exhibit electrophoretic heterogenic mobility and can be found in the $alpha_1$, $alpha_2$, beta, and gamma regions in serum protein electrophoresis. Much like other active protein systems (for example, coagulation factors), the proteins interact in a specific cascading sequence. The result of this cascading activation is significant biologic activity. The complexity is required for integration with other systems and homeostatic control.

Table 15. Characteristics and nomenclature of the complement system*

Component	Synonym	Electrophoretic mobility	Mol wt	Normal serum concentration (ng/ml)
C1q		Gamma	4×10^5	120-200
C1r	C1 esterase (C1q, C1r, C1s)	Beta	1.68×10^5	60-80
C1s		$Alpha_2$	7.9×10^4	30-60
C2	C3 convertase (C2, C4)	Beta	1.17×10^5	20-40
C4		Beta	2.4×10^5	170-200
C3	β-1-C-globulin	Beta	1.85×10^5	800-1500
C5		Beta	1.25×10^5	60-90
C6	Trimolecular complex (C5, C6, C7)	Beta		40-80
C7		Beta		40-80
C8		Beta	1.5×10^5	1-10
C9		$Alpha_2$	7.9×10^4	1-10

*Modification of a report by The World Health Organization, 1968.

Each component of the complement system is designated numerically according to its order of discovery. Note that C4 emerged in the second position of activation, that is, C1, C4, C2, C3, C5, C6, C7, C8, C9. It was later shown that in reality C1 was composed of three types of subunits, C1q, C1r, and C1s, and possibly a recently described C1t. Subunits and fragments are designated with a lowercase letter. Inactive forms are indicated with "i," for example, C2i. Table 15, released by the World Health Organization in 1968, indicates the suggested nomenclature and some of the known characteristics of the complement system. Several organs have been implicated as possible sources of complement synthesis including the liver.

Activation

The prime directive of the complement system is to defend the integrity of the body. While the responsibility of antibody is to recognize and bind antigen, the role of complement is to attack and destroy. Antibody searches out and identifies foreign substances, while complement destroys the foreign substance. The reaction of antibody with antigen gives specificity to complement action. Binding of antigen with antibody evidently causes a conformational change to occur in the Fc region of immunoglobulins. The molecular shift causes exposure of certain chemical groups in the C_H2 domain. These groups can be recognized by $C1_q$ component of complement, resulting in binding. The C_H2 region of all immunoglobulins is not capable of complement binding, rather only those immunoglobulins that play an active role in infectious disease immunity, IgG_1, IgG_2, IgG_3, and IgM. Activation appears related not only to the type of immunoglobulins but also to the number. Studies have shown that a minimum of four heavy chains in close association is necessary for complement activation. This last restriction in part accounts for the greater efficiency of IgM than IgG in activating complement. Two adjacent IgG molecules would be necessary to activate complement while

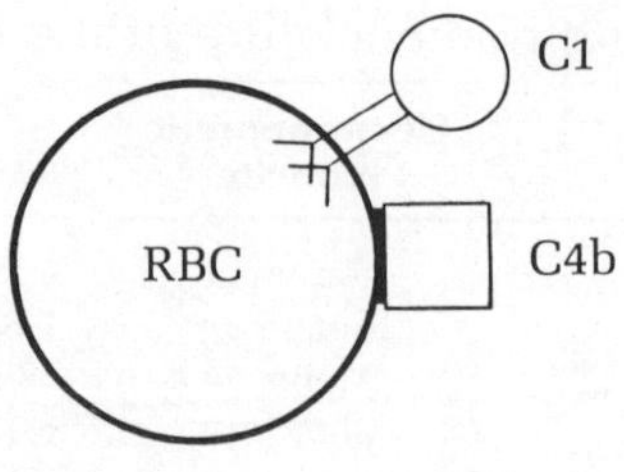

Fig. 7-1. Binding of two IgG molecules in close approximation. Cellular antigen acts as receptor for C1q, leading to assembly of active $\overline{C1}$. Enzymatic action on C4 results in C4b binding to cell surface receptor.

one IgM antibody would suffice. Excessive antigen concentrations would tend to reduce the possibility of two IgG antibodies reacting at adjacent sites. For this reason, complement activation is sensitive to, and inhibited by, postzone.

The activation of each component is indicated by a bar, that is, $\overline{C1}$. The C1 component, like many other complement components, is considered to be a proenzyme. This proenzyme is composed of three subunits C1q, C1r, and C1s. The subunits of C1 are assembled at the site of the binding of C1q. The subunits are held together via chelation with the calcium ion. Antibody identifies the target and then acts as a receptor for C1q, which is followed by the assembly of C1 as shown in equation 7-1.

$$\mathrm{Ag}\Big\langle{}^{\mathrm{Ab}}_{\mathrm{Ab}} \;+\; {}^{\mathrm{q}}_{\mathrm{r}}\Big\rangle \mathrm{C1\text{---}s} \quad \mathrm{AgAb}\overline{\mathrm{C1}} \qquad \textbf{(Eq. 7-1)}$$

This first major event in complement activation is called recognition. The activated C1 then proceeds to cleave C4 molecules into two fragments, C4a and C4b. The C4a fragment is small and is rapidly lost and inactivated in the blood. The C4b fragment has an active site capable of binding to the surface of cells. After C4b is bound to the cell surface, C2 is absorbed to it and then cleaved by the neighboring active C1, C1 esterase (note Fig. 7-1). The cleavage of C2 produces two fragments, C2a and C2b. The C2a component then binds to C4b resulting in a new active enzyme, C3 convertase. As shown in equation 7-2, the natural substrate for C3 convertase is C3.

$$\mathrm{C2} \xrightarrow{\overline{\mathrm{C14b}}} \mathrm{Ag}\overline{\mathrm{AbC14b2a}} + \mathrm{2b} \qquad \textbf{(Eq. 7-2)}$$

As can be seen in equation 7-3, C3 convertase is a proteolytic enzyme capable of catalyzing a reaction that leads to the production of a shower of C3 fragments.

$$\mathrm{C3} \xrightarrow{\mathrm{AgAb}\overline{\mathrm{C14b2a}}} \mathrm{C3a} + \mathrm{C3b} \qquad \textbf{(Eq. 7-3)}$$

The smaller C3 fragment, C3a, is released and is a mediator of inflammation as will be discussed below. The second C3 fragment, C3b, binds to cell surface receptors. The C3b with its neighboring bound C14b2a proceeds to cleave C5 as shown in equation 7-4.

$$C5 \xrightarrow{AgAbC\overline{14b2a3b}} C5a + C5b \quad \textbf{(Eq. 7-4)}$$

Splitting of C5 initiates the attack phase of complement activation. The C5a fragment is released and also is a mediator of inflammation. The C5b fragment has two possible fates. It may bind to C14b2a3b and proceed to bind C6 then diffuse away or it may remain bound. C6 plays the role of stabilizer for the complement complex. Binding of C7 generates a reactive site that is capable of attachment to the cell's membrane. It appears that C8 combines with C5b and then C9 binds to C8.

Activation of alternate pathway

Studies have shown the existence of what might be considered a more natural pathway of activation. This alternate pathway is less specific than the classical pathway. Activation of the alternate pathway is the result of any circumstance that generates enzymes capable of acting on C3 and C5. Various kinds of polysaccharides when incubated with normal serum can activate complement via this mechanism. These polysaccharides are frequently associated with bacterial membranes and bacterial endotoxins. Clearly there would be a major physiologic advantage to this type of nonspecific activation. This type of activation can be set in motion prior to the induction of a humoral immune response. Activation via the alternate pathway results in a bypass of C1, C4, and C2 and starts with cleavage of C3. Even though alternate pathway complement activation has poor lytic activity, the ensuing activation steps lead to the release of factors that attract white cells (chemotactic factors) and cause the release of pharmacologic mediators of inflammation (anaphylatoxins). The effect, in total, is to aid the body in bringing about the elimination of the offending agents. The factors capable of activating the alternate pathway include inulin, zymosan, bacterial polysaccharide, aggregated immunoglobulins, IgG_4, IgA, and IgE. Through a still ill-defined system, the initiation factors act via the properdin system and generate an active proteolytic enzyme. This system is composed of properdin and factors A,B,O° (note equations 7-5 and 7-6).

$$\text{Initiation factors} \xrightarrow{\text{Properdin system}} \text{C3 activator} \quad \textbf{(Eq. 7-5)}$$

$$C3 \xrightarrow[\text{Activator}]{\text{C3}} C3b + C3a \quad \textbf{(Eq. 7-6)}$$

Biologic activity of complement

The most commonly studied activity of complement is lysis. After years of study the exact mechanism is still not totally understood. The cells attacked by complement have been shown via electron microscopy and scanning electromicroscopy to be speckled with holes. It is likely that the passage of ions out of the cell and water into the cell is the cause of cellular swelling and finally lysis. This is best shown with red blood cells, which upon attack release their hemoglobin, producing the typical ghost cell. But the question of how the holes were made remains a mystery. An early theory proposed that late-acting complement components served as enzymes that were capable of "drilling" holes through membranes. A more current theory states that late-acting components arrange hydrophobic groups in such a way that they are capable of dissolving away the membrane surface in a detergent-like action. A difficulty with both the above theories arises from the fact we now know that cell membranes more resemble a "lipid sea" than a solid wall. If this is fact, then how can we account for the stability of the "drilled holes" in a fluid matrix? A possible answer comes from a theory that the late-acting components bind to the cell membrane in such a way that they produce a stable protein "donut."

Several other nonlytic, biologic effects occur when complement is activated by either pathway. The C3a and C5a fragments, for example, mediate the release of histamine and other powerful pharmacologic agents from leukocytes and mast cells. These agents are capable of increasing vascular permeability and causing smooth muscle contraction, which results in the many symptoms of allergy. Increased vascular permeability permits penetration of white blood cells into the surrounding tissues. Chemotactic factors (C5a, C5b67) attract cells through vessel walls to the site of complement activation. Historically the role of complement activation has been thought to be primarily implicated in the elimination of cellular invaders. Recent discoveries of C3b receptors on B cells and macrophages have aroused new speculation on the role of complement. Activation of complement by immune complexes could result in the attachment of C3b to the complex. Receptors on phagocytes and B cells for C3b would then aid phagocytosis and antibody response. The sequel to this theory is that activation via the alternate pathway may actually promote induction of a cellular and humoral response.

Interactions

Future studies in complement research will surely elaborate a finely tuned system capable of interacting with many physiologic processes. The interaction of complement with the coagulation of blood has had much attention and is worked out in some detail. Normal clotting requires C6, but aside from this a more complex system exists. Factor XII (coagulation system), the Hageman factor, plays a pivotal role. Factor XII performs at least three major functions:

1. Initiates the clotting
2. Initiates dissolution of the clot via activation of plasmin
3. Mediates the release of kinins (Fig. 7-2)

If, for example, an object broke the skin and entered a vessel, activation of Factor XII indirectly would begin the repair of the vascular disturbance through the clotting mechanism. Meanwhile, Factor XII activation of plasmin would in-

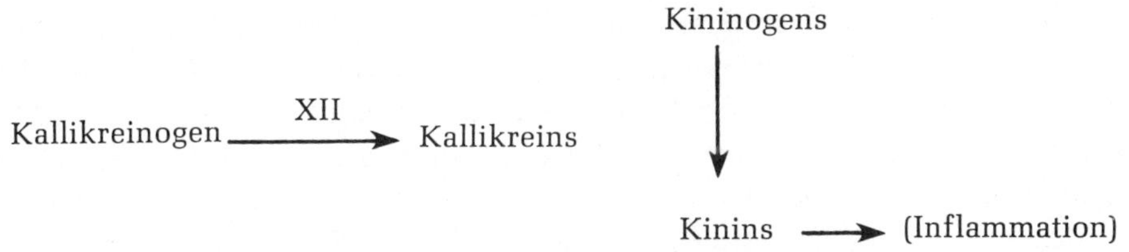

Fig. 7-2. Role of factor XII in kinin release.

itiate fibrinolysis to prevent excessive intravascular coagulation. Plasmin also is able to activate C1s and promote the complement cascade as well as directly cleaving C3. Once activated the complement system may indeed be immediately responsible for the defense of the body.

Regulatory mechanisms

The powers of this system must be controlled. Imagine the result of a cascading and amplifying complement system without control. This system is far from totally understood, but some basic observations explain how activation and the ensuing response are localized. A key regulatory effect is obtained via the limited stability of complement components, fragment, and newly formed binding sites. For example, C1, C3, C4, and C5 have extremely short active stages and rapidly lose all known activity. The $\overline{C4b2a}$ complex has a 10-minute half-life at 37° C. This limited lifetime phenomenon serves to restrict the response to the area where complement activation is occurring, thereby preventing the effects of complement activity at distant sites.

Inhibitors and inactivators of many complement components have been demonstrated in normal human serum. The best known inhibitor is C1 esterase inhibitor (C1 INH). C1 INH also inhibits kinin formation, Factor XII, plasmin, and coagulation Factor IX. Inhibitors for C3b and C4b have also been described, and deficiencies have been shown to be related to increased susceptibility to infection. Inhibitors to C3 and C6 act on bound activated complement. An antibody to certain molecular groups of C3 and C4, known as immune conglutinin, inhibits immune adherence. Proteolytic enzymes such as trypsin also may aid in regulating complement activity.

Immunopathology and complement

The most common physiologic problems related to complement are due to immune complex activation of the complement system. The formation of immune complexes, particularly in antigen excess, allows the soluble complex to permeate extravascular tissue. Once into the tissue, an in vivo system comparable to gel diffusion is set up. As antibody concentration increases antigen-antibody precipitation and complement activation can occur. Complement activation may occur through the classical or alternate pathway and results in release of complement fragments. Factors such as C3a and C5a increase vascular permeability, while C5a and C5b67 are chemotactic. The C3b fragments bind to receptors on cells and immune complexes aiding phagocytosis. The result of this sequence of events is an inflammatory response with a massive infiltration of phagocytic cells. The immune system has efficiently developed an attack to eliminate the offending agents. However, the high number of phagocytic cells in the area releases lysoenzymes into the tissue causing autodestruction of tissue. Further activation of the complement system can proceed to initiate clotting leading to thrombosis. This disastrous sequence of events occurs in serum sickness, immune complex diseases, and certain types of nephritis.

A serious difficulty arising from the activation of complement is seen in what is known as cytotoxic reactions. The damage in this type of hypersensitivity is due to the misdirected lytic activity of complement rather than the effect of component mediators. Cytotoxic reaction can be due to antibody reaction with foreign cells, for example, transfusion reactions, altered antigens (keflin alteration), red blood cell antigens, new antigens (viral association with surface antigens), or measles.

The components of the complement system have been isolated and purified. These recent advances have allowed the development of specific antisera that enable the detection of absolute and relative deficiencies of complement. With these advances, laboratories are detecting deficiencies in most components. The most prevalent and therefore important has been the deficiency of C1 esterase inhibitor (autosomal dominant trait). These individuals develop massive areas of swelling, and the condition is known as hereditary angioedema. Deficiencies in the properdin system have been reported, and these people are susceptible to severe recurrent infections. Some complement deficiencies show no signs and symptoms.

EVALUATION OF THE COMPLEMENT SYSTEM

Assessment of complement components is gaining interest in most clinical laboratories. This is happening for at least two reasons:

1. Increased understanding of the implications of complement activity
2. Development of specific antisera

With specific antisera it is possible to measure complement protein via RID or EID. The clinical laboratory is able to measure C1q, C3, and C4 in the classical pathway and Factor B and properdin in the alternate pathway. Complement is frequently evaluated to identify the complement-depleted individual. This situation may be due to increased utilization in hyperimmune active conditions as is seen in patients with systemic lupus erythematosus, acute glomerulonephritis, and chronic glomerulonephritis. The level of complement activity often has a close inverse correlation with disease process activity. Since complement components are considered to be acute reactant proteins, elevations would expectedly be encountered frequently. Complement profiling has recently been shown to be of diagnostic value (Table 16). Simultaneous determinations of C3, C4, and Fac-

Table 16. Complement profile in SLE and AGN

	C3	C4	Factor B
SLE	↓	↓	↓
AGN	↓	↑	↓

NOTE: SLE = systemic lupus erythematosus (nephritis); AGN = acute glomerulonephritis.

Table 17. Simplified complement assay procedure outline

Tube	Dilution (7.0 pH buffer)	2% sRBC	Incubation (30 min)	Hemolysis (%)
1	1:1	1	37° C	80
2	1:2	1	37° C	80
3	1:4	1	37° C	80
4	1:8	1	37° C	60
5	1:16	1	37° C	50
6	1:32	1	37° C	30
7	1:64	1	37° C	10
8	1:128	1	37° C	0
9	Buffer	1	37° C	0
10	H_2O	1	37° C	100

tor B provide the diagnostician with a useful aid to distinguish acute glomerulonephritis from the nephritis of systemic lupus erythematosus.

Complement hemolytic activity

Kits are commercially available for RID testing of C1q, C3, C4, Factor B, properdin, and C1 esterase inhibition. The principal methods and limitations of RID discussed in Chapter 5 apply to the testing of the complement protein. Because complement is a system with specific activity, RID testing has predictable inherent problems. In RID the laboratory tests immunospecificity of complement not its activity. For this reason there is still some interest in measuring hemolytic activity.

Principles. In the first step of the assay red blood cells are mixed with complement-deficient specific antiserum. This results in antibody binding to red blood cell antigenic sites; however, since no complement is available, lysis does not occur (equation 7-7). These sensitized, antibody-coated red blood cells then can be used to detect complement as shown in equation 7-8. When the patient serum is serially diluted and separate aliquots are added to the sensitized red blood cells, lysis will occur only until the serum complement is diluted to some critically low level.

$$\text{Anti-RBC} + \text{RBC} \rightarrow \text{Coated Ab-RBC} \qquad \textbf{(Eq. 7-7)}$$

$$\text{Serum-C} + \text{Ab-RBC} \rightarrow \text{Hemolysis} \qquad \textbf{(Eq. 7-8)}$$

To increase the precision of complement-hemolytic assays all reagents must be carefully standardized. Most laboratories report complement activity in C_H50 units. This unit is based on the dilution that lyses 50% of the red blood cells available. Some procedure employs colorimetric analysis of supernatant hemoglobin to determine this 50% point.

Methodology. In the simplified assay described in Table 17, the patient's serum is serially diluted with buffered saline solution. Equal volumes of sensitized red blood cells are added to each tube. Tube no. 9 contains only buffer and cells and is a negative control. Tube no. 10 has distilled water and cells and will demonstrates 100% lysis. After 30 minutes of incubation in a 37° C water bath, the tubes are centrifuged and the absorbance of the supernatants are read photometrically at 415 nm. The absorbance (A) of the dilutions and the 100% lysis tube are used to calculate % hemolysis, as shown in equation 7-9.

$$\frac{\text{A Tube 10}}{\text{A Tube X}} \times 100 = \%\ \text{Hemolysis} \qquad \textbf{(Eq. 7-9)}$$

Interpretation. Total complement activity is depressed in systemic lupus erythematosus. It is also low in chronic and acute glomerulonephritis and in autoimmune hemolytic anemia. Certain kidney and liver diseases can produce lowered hemolytic complement activity by way of a depressed rate of synthesis of particular components. It is imperative to adhere strictly to the procedure in all complement activity assays. Not only is complement a protein susceptible to variation in environment, but the patient's serum may demonstrate anticomplement activity. Variations in the red blood cell suspension the antibody used to sensitize the red blood cells, pH of the buffer, and the ionic strength of the buffer all may affect total activity. All reagents must be standardized and tested through the proper use of controls. The assay just described primarily tests the classical pathway and fails to detect problems in the properdinalternate pathway. The assay does provide a means to screen all of the components of the classical pathway, since all are necessary for hemolysis.

X

Complement fixation tests

Principles and limitations. Complement fixation (CF) tests are sensitive and versatile assays used to detect and measure either antigen or antibody. The principle of the CF test is based on the fact that certain immune complexes are able to bind or fix complement. In such binding the immune complex consumes available complement. Sensitized red blood cells added to thc complement-depleted serum would not lyse, for complement is fixed to the immune complex. In Table 18 this reaction is seen in Tube no. 1. If homologous antigen and antibody are present, then complement is in effect removed from the test system and therefore is not available to lyse sensitized red blood cells as shown in equation 7-10. Equations 7-11 and 7-12 and Tubes 2 and 3 of Table 18 demonstrate the inability of antigen alone or antibody to fix complement.

Q.4

Table 18. Outline of possible complement fixation reactions

	Antigen	Antibody	GPC	sRBC	Hemolysis	Test
Tube 1	+	+	+	+	−	+
Tube 2	−	+	+	+	+	−
Tube 3	+	−	+	+	+	−

NOTE: GPC = guinea pig complement; sRBC = sheep red blood cells coated with rabbit antibody.

$$\left.\begin{matrix}\text{Ag}\\ \text{Ab}\end{matrix}\right\rangle \text{C} + \text{sRBC} \rightarrow \text{No hemolysis} \qquad \textbf{(Eq. 7-10)}$$

$$\text{Ag} + \text{C} + \text{sRBC} \rightarrow \text{Hemolysis} \qquad \textbf{(Eq. 7-11)}$$

$$\text{Ab} + \text{C} + \text{sRBC} \rightarrow \text{Hemolysis} \qquad \textbf{(Eq. 7-12)}$$

Each antigen-antibody complex is capable of fixing only a limited amount of complement. If an excess of complement is present, then lysis may occur even though the antigen has reacted with antibody. Because of this, the potency of the guinea pig (GP) complement used in the assay must be carefully assessed. Once the potency is determined, the GP complement must be diluted to the appropriate concentration. The patient's serum should be heat inactivated and tested for anticomplementary activity. Many patients, such as those with rheumatoid arthritis, may have immune complexes present in their serum. These immune complexes may bind available complement and indicate a false positive test. An anticomplementary control need only contain patient sample, GP complement, and sensitized red blood cells. If the serum is anticomplementary, it will nonspecifically absorb complement, and the sensitized red blood cells will not lyse.

Viral studies. The CF test can be and is employed in the diagnosis of many viral and fungal diseases. The complexity and time requirements of the assay discourage the use of these tests in many laboratories. The availability of RID for many of the studies precludes the use of the CF test. Large viral serology laboratories frequently utilize the CF assay to test paired serum samples against a battery of viral and fungal antigens, such as influenza A and B, mumps, herpes, and adenoviruses. A partial list of diseases in which an antibody response may be detected by complement fixation assay follows:

- Mumps
- Influenza A and B
- Parainfluenza
- Respiratory syncytial virus
- Encephalitis
- Lymphocytic choriomeningitis
- Coxsackievirus
- Measles
- Rubella
- Cytomegalovirus
- Colorado tick fever

Most viral CF tests require the use of antigens prepared in human cell culture. The species specificity of many viral organisms frequently results in contamination of the viral antigens with cell culture antigens. Another problem seen in CF testing of viral antigens is due to the ubiquitous nature of many viruses. Most individuals are left with a low titer to many of these viruses. For this reason it is almost impossible to interpret single sample assays. Clinically useful data are derived when blood samples are obtained during both the acute and convalescent stages of illness. Generally the popularity of the CF test is waning, partly because of the increased use of newer, more rapid techniques such as radioimmunoassays.

READINGS AND RESOURCES

Alper, C. A., and Rosen, F. S.: Genetic aspects of the complement system, Adv. Immunol. **14:**251, 1975.

Augener, W., Grey, H. M., and Cooper, N. R.: The reaction of monomeric and aggregated immunoglobulins with C1, Immunochemistry **6:**461, 1969.

Carlin, H.: Problem clinic: complement, Hosp. Top. **41,** August, 1972.

Kohler, P. F., and Muller-Eberhard, H. J.: Immunochemical quantitation of the third, fourth and fifth components of human complement: concentrations in the serum of healthy adults, J. Immunol. **99:**1211, 1967.

Kolb, W. P., et al.: Molecular analysis of membrane attack mechanisms of complement, J. Exp. Med. **135:**549, 1972.

Lepow, I. H.: Biologically active fragments of complement. In Amos, D. B., editor: Progress in immunology, New York, 1972, Academic Press, Inc.

Mayer, M. M.: The complement system, Sci. Am. **229:**54, 1973.

Muller-Eberhard, H. J.: Complement, Ann. Rev. Biochem. **44:**697, 1975.

Ritzman, S. E., and Daniels, J. C.: Serum protein abnormalities, Boston, 1975, Little, Brown & Co.

Rose, N. R., and Bigazzi, P. E., editors: Methods in immunodiagnosis, New York, 1973, John Wiley & Sons, Inc.

Rose, N. R., and Friedman, H., editors: Manual of clinical immunology, A.S.M. Washington, D.C., 1976.

Scornik, J. C.: Complement dependent immunoglobulin G receptor function in lymphoid cells, Science **192:**563, 1976.

CHAPTER 8

Neutralization

The interaction of biologically active antigens with homologous antibody sometimes yields a loss in the antigen's biologic activity. The term "neutralization" is used to generally describe this type of immune reaction. Some immunologists classify the neutralization reaction among the most sensitive and specific of the immunoassays. Despite the sensitivity and specificity of neutralization tests, these assays are infrequently used. The major limitation is inherent in the definition of neutralization, that is, that the antigen must have biologically detectable activity.

IN VIVO NEUTRALIZATION REACTION

Antibody response to active molecules occurs in vivo and is responsible for the signs and symptoms of many disorders. The induction of these antibodies in some individuals is difficult to explain. However, the presence of these antibodies may be due to autoimmune disorders, transfusion reactions, drug reactions, or cross-reactive antibodies. Insulin resistance in certain diabetics appears to be due to the presence of neutralizing antibodies. Antibodies to clotting factors have been associated with several disorders including systemic lupus erythematosus, hypergammaglobulinemia, and tuberculosis. These coagulation-factor antibodies sometimes result in bleeding disorders. Hemophiliacs who genetically lack factor VIII may develop neutralizing antibodies that hinder factor VIII replacement therapy. Certain patients develop antibodies to intrinsic factor, a factor necessary for the absorption of vitamin B_{12}. B_{12} is required in the normal maturation of the erythrocyte. A deficiency in B_{12}, caused by the neutralization of intrinsic factor, eventually leads to a macrocytic hypochromic anemia. Apparently, infertility may be due to the presence of neutralizing antibody against spermatozoa in either the male or female. These few examples serve to exemplify the potential effect of antibodies that are capable of neutralizing biologically active molecules.

Mechanisms

The mechanism of neutralization presumably varies from antigen to antigen. However, certain generalizations are in order. It is known that binding of antibody with antigen can result in a conformational change in both molecules. This new conformation may totally lack activity, or the activity could be markedly curtailed. Another possibility is that binding of antibody may occur at or near the active site of the antigen. Binding at or near the active site could sterically block activity. Antibody binding could change a necessary surface charge or activate the complement system and yield destruction.

IN VITRO NEUTRALIZATION REACTION

Mechanisms

The in vitro application of this phenomenon has always been fraught with problems. To develop a neutralization assay for commercial use one needs an unlimited supply of active antigen. The antigen must be used in an assay environment that does not induce loss of activity. Among other difficulties, the antigen must have measurable or at least detectable activity. Neutralization assays tend to be qualitative and are highly susceptible to false positive results; that is, any situation that leads to neutralization of antigen activity may be interpreted as caused by antibody. The major advantage of the neutralization assay is that neutralizing antibodies are extremely sensitive and specific, even though most assays have inherent problems. Several useful and valuable clinical applications are discussed in the following sections.

Influenza

The body normally responds to an infection with a virus in many ways such as by way of production of interferon (a nonimmune viral inhibitor), antibody, and cellular responses. The antibodies may be of several classes and obviously produced from many clones of cells. These antibodies are normally directed at a variety of antigenic determinants, some internal and some external. When influenza is the causative agent of infection, there are four major antigens of clinical interest to the laboratory. These antigens are:

1. M (matrix)
2. NP (nucleoprotein)
3. NA (neuramidinase)
4. HA (hemagglutinin)

Most assays for influenza employ at least one of these antigens.

The simplest viral neutralization test is sometimes called the animal protection test. This assay makes use of the fact that certain animals are highly susceptible to various viral agents. If the viral suspension is treated with the serum of a patient with neutralizing antibodies prior to animal injection, then infectivity is lost. Protective antibody is therefore measured through a decrease in morbidity. Similar neutralization studies are performed in a wide variety of systems, for example, inhibition of cytopathic effect on tissue culture, reduction in plaque-forming colonies on each egg allantoic membrane, and so on. The level of protection is determined by serially diluting the patient's serum prior to mixing with the virus preparation. In general, viral-neutralizing antibodies are persistent and may be detectable in a serum sample months and even years after infection. Single determinations of protective-neutralizing antibody titer are of little value. Significance is obtained via simultaneous testing of acute and convalescent serum followed by careful evaluation of changing titers.

Principles. Many viruses are capable of agglutinating red blood cells. The agglutinating power of these viruses is an example of biologic activity, and this activity can be inhibited by certain antibodies. Specific sites on the viral particles are capable of interacting with mucoprotein receptors on the red blood cells and other cell surfaces. The interaction of receptor sites and virion leads to visible agglutination of red blood cells. A viral enzyme neuramidinase then cleaves the bridge between the virus and cell, releasing both into the solution. In the neutralization assay for influenza, the laboratory takes advantage of this hemagglutination reaction.

The viral site where attachment occurs is antigenic and is referred to as the hemagglutinin (HA), and antibodies to HA can be tested for in a very sensitive hemagglutination-inhibition (HI) assay. The neutralization test is simple, requires no elaborate equipment, glassware, or skills, and is readily adaptable to microtechnique.

Methodology. Mucoproteins present in the serum of patients may inhibit hemagglutination by binding viral HA. For this reason the serum being tested is treated with neuramidinase prior to assaying. For each patient two sets of tubes are appropriately labeled with type A and type B. A serum sample in each set is serially twofold diluted in an appropriate diluent. Standardized suspensions of each virus preparation are added to the appropriate set of tubes, for example, equal amounts of type A suspension to each tube labeled A and equal amounts of B suspension to each tube labeled B. (Viral antigens are commercially available.) The mixtures are agitated and incubated for 30 minutes at room temperature. A constant amount of a standardized red blood cell suspension is added to each tube after incubation. The rack of tubes is incubated until all cells settle to the bottom of the tubes. Agglutinated and nonagglutinated cells settle into unique and readily distinguishable patterns as shown in Fig. 8-1. The HI titer is reported as the highest dilution completely inhibiting viral red blood cell agglutination.

Interpretation. The World Health Organization suggests that a fourfold change in HI titer may be considered significant. As mentioned previously, HI antibodies may persist for years, but persistent titers change little over a 2- to 3-week period. The success of the HI assays depends on many factors, including proper standardization of red blood cell viral suspensions as well as proper handling of patient serum. As shown in Table 19, appropriate controls must be run in each batch to assure reliability. A control must be included for each patient to test for nonspecific red blood cell–agglutinating antibodies. If present, red blood cell agglutinins would not be inhibited by neutralizing antibodies and therefore may indicate false negative results. A 50% suspension of red blood cells can be used to absorb these serum agglutinins prior to retesting. A known (previously titrated) reference control serum must be titrated separately with type A and type B influenza virus. The reference control monitors many parameters including red blood cell and viral suspensions, technical skills, and interpretation. In one tube a red blood cell suspension with no other reagents can be used as a visual comparator for no agglutination or a positive reaction.

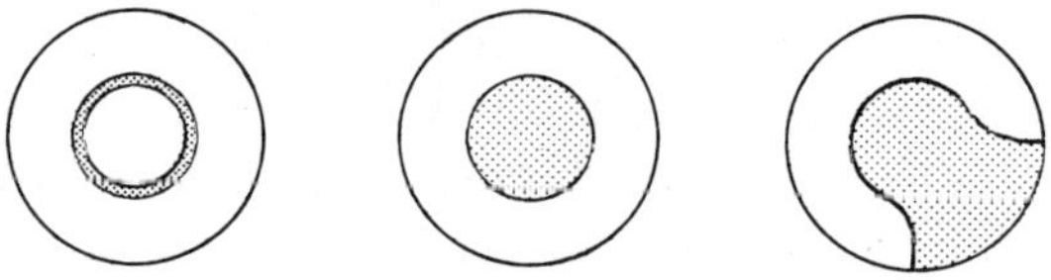

Fig. 8-1. Erythrocyte settling patterns in hemagglutination assay for influenza antibodies. **A,** Completely agglutinated cells. **B,** Nonagglutinated cells. **C,** Incompletely agglutinated cells.

Table 19. Outline of complement fixation assay for antibody to influenza A and B

Tube set	Neuramidinase-treated serum (patient or control)	Virus A suspension	Virus B suspension	RBC suspension	Expected results
(1) Nonspecific agglutination—control	+	0	0	+	No agglutination
(2) Influenza A—patient	+	+	0	+	Dilution equals titer
(3) Influenza B—patient test	+	0	+	+	Dilution equals titer
(4) Positive agglutination—control A serum (ref)	+	+	0	+	Within one dilution of known titer
(5) Positive agglutination—control B serum (ref)	+	0	+	+	Within one dilution of known titer
(6) Virus agglutinating ability—control A	0	+	0	+	Agglutination
(7) Virus agglutinating ability—control B	0	0	+	+	Agglutination
(8) Cell—control	0	0	0	+	No agglutination

NOTE: + indicates the addition of reagent; 0 indicates the absence of the reagent; ref. indicates an assayed reference sample with a statistically evaluated known titer.

Spermatozoa immobilization

Principles. It has been shown that approximately 15% of the couples in the United States are afflicted with infertility. Many of these individuals, both male or female, have developed neutralizing antibodies that may be responsible for the infertility. These individuals can be identified readily by two tests, the spermatozoa agglutination test or the spermatozoa immobilization test. Laboratories seriously interested in identifying antispermatozoa antibodies utilize both assays. The principle of both assays is relatively simple; however, the discussion to follow is limited to the immobilization test.

Presumably the cause for infertility may be that neutralizing antibody is capable of halting the forward movement of spermatozoa. In vitro studies using rabbit antisera prepared via immunizations with human spermatozoa have demonstrated this immobilization and have shown the reaction to be complement dependent.

Methodology. Fresh motile human sperm is diluted with buffer to yield a final concentration of approximately 60×10^6/ml. Both the male and female serum samples as well as the positive and negative controls are heat inactivated. The patient sample, the positive control, and the negative control are added to the appropriately labeled tubes. Guinea pig complement and freshly diluted spermatozoa are added to each tube. The mixture is incubated at 37° C for 1 hour and then microscopically viewed for motility. The positive control may be antisera prepared in rabbit.

Interpretation. Initial screening of patients is performed with undiluted serum specimens; however, a high percentage of false positives may be encountered. All positive samples should be titrated. The end point of this assay is the dilution that results in at least a 50% reduction in the total number of motile spermatozoa (50% of normal control number). In one study, 18% of the infertile couples (N = 74) demonstrated spermatozoa antibodies via either the agglutination test or the immobilization assay. It was not possible to detect this antibody in any of 83 pregnant women.

Coagulation factor inhibitors

Principles. Patients with congenital coagulation factor deficiencies, autoimmune disorders, and a variety of other disorders have been shown to acquire inhibitors to the normal clotting system of the body. Some of these inhibitors have clearly been shown to be antibody, while others are highly suspect. Before discussing immune coagulopathies and the assays used to test for them, it is necessary to briefly review the normal coagulation scheme. As shown in the boxed material (p. 124) at least thirteen factors are necessary for normal coagulation.

In a much simplified fashion, Fig. 8-2 illustrates the four major phases of normal coagulation and how the various factors interact. The intrinsic (plasma-activated) pathway leads to activation of each factor through a cascading interaction. This cascade leads to the final conversion of soluble fibrinogen to insoluble fibrin.

Coagulation factors and synonyms

Factor	Synonym
I	Fibrinogen
II	Prothrombin
III	Thromboplastin
IV	Calcium
V	Labile factor
VI	
VII	Proconvertin
VIII	Antihemophilic factor
IX	Christmas factor
X	Stuart-Prower factor
XI	Plasma thromboplastin antecedent
XII	Hageman factor
XIII	Fibrin-stabilizing factor

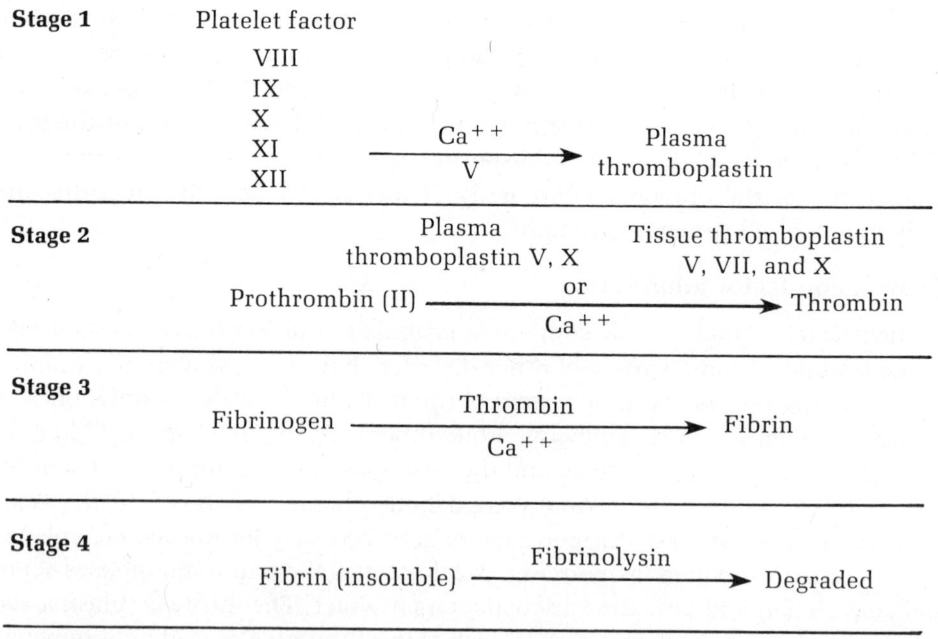

Fig. 8-2. Simplified coagulation scheme.

The formation of fibrin provides a matrix or network that serves as the foundation for the forming clot. Thromboplastin released from tissue damage (extrinsic pathway) bypasses phase one, inactivation of prothrombin. The clinical hematology laboratory utilizes many tests to monitor the coagulatory capacity of the body. The prothrombin time (PT) and the partial thromboplastin time (PTT) have become the most popular of these assays. As shown in the boxed material below, the PT and PTT are sensitive to deficiences in activity of most coagulation factors. The basic principle of most of the coagulation tests is based on the fact that coagulation-deficient plasma is not able to form a clot in the normal time interval. If blood is collected in a citrated container, calcium is effectively removed, hence the coagulation process halts. However, the addition of calcium plus certain of the coagulation factors allows screening for deficiency of those factors not added. The unit of measure is usually time, and the end point is estimated utilizing the formation of mucus-like fibrin during clot formation. A patient with a factor deficiency or a factor inhibitor will likely show a prolongation of either or both the PT and PTT. For example, a deficiency or inhibitor to factor VII will probably result in a prolonged PT and a normal PTT when tested.

Acquired inhibitors to factors I, V, VIII, IX, X, XI, and XII have been reported. Frequently, acquisition of these inhibitors follows transfusions, antibiotic therapy, or development of autoimmune disease. The fundamental distinguishing characteristic of the acquired inhibitor is that the inhibitor plasma cannot be normalized by the addition of coagulation factors. For example, a patient with a deficiency of factor VIII (hemophiliac) will, when tested, demonstrate a prolonged PTT. If the deficient plasma is mixed with factor VIII or even mixed with normal plasma, the prolonged PTT should be corrected. However, the patient with an inhibitor to factor VIII will not demonstrate this correction when the plasma is mixed with factor VIII or when it is mixed with normal plasma. It would appear that, like other tests already discussed, the previous assay is a typical neutralization test. The antigens are clotting factors and the biologic activity is clotting. The inhibitor is an acquired antibody capable of being assayed via a classical neutralization test.

Methodology. The patient sample is first screened via the PTT and PT for coagulopathy. If an unexplained prolongation of the PTT or PT is noted, one may proceed to check for the presence of inhibitors. This is accomplished by mixing

Factors assayed in the PT and PTT

Assay	Coagulation factors tested
Prothrombin time (PT)	II, V, VII, X
Partial thromboplastin time (PTT)	XIII, IX, X, XI, XII

Table 20. Typical results of coagulation inhibitor studies

	PT/PTT	PT/PTT after addition of normal plasma
Normal patient	Normal	
Factor-deficient patient	Abnormal	Corrected
Factor-inhibitor patient	Abnormal	Abnormal

equal amounts of normal citrated plasma with the abnormal patient plasma. After mixing the PT and PTT are repeated.

Interpretation. The typical results for the previous procedure on a normal patient, a patient with a factor deficiency, and a patient with an inhibitor are noted in Table 20. If the addition of normal citrated plasma does not correct the coagulopathy, then it is likely an inhibitor is present. The identity of the inhibitor must be found through further assays. Many of the inhibitors so far studied have been shown to be immunoglobulins. For example, the inhibitor to factor IX is stable over a wide range of temperature and pH and on column fractionation was shown to be in the IgG fraction. Treatment of the factor IX inhibitor plasma with anti-IgG resulted in loss of inhibitory activity.

Antistreptolysin O (ASO)

Principles. Damage to kidney or cardiac tissue frequently follows infection with certain streptococcal organisms. The tissue damage appears to be due to antibodies that are cytotoxic to these tissues. It seems that these antibodies may be directed at bacterial antigens absorbed to the cell surface or that the antibodies may be cross-reactive. Another theory holds that *de novo* antigens are created by the bacteria-cell complex. In this discussion we are most interested in post-streptococcal acute glomerulonephritis. This type of nephritis is associated with infections with only a few strains of group A beta-hemolytic streptococci.

On infecting man these streptococcal organisms elaborate several important antigens, both intracellular and extracellular (which may be toxins, bacterial poisons, or enzymes, and so on). These antigens are utilized in many diagnostic immunoassays. The most popularly used antigens are extracellular soluble bacterial products such as streptolysin, deoxyribonuclease-B (DNase-B), hyaluronidase, nicotinamide-adenine dinucleotidase, and streptokinase. The neutralization test employing streptolysin O, an enzyme like toxin, is probably the most frequently used test.

Streptolysin O is a protein produced by Lancefield group A streptococci and by a few strains of group C and G streptococci. Streptolysin O is inactive in the oxidized state and has lytic activity in the reduced state. Streptolysin O is capable of lysing both white and red blood cells. Streptolysin O is susceptible to oxidation in room air and therefore must be protected from oxidation. In the ASO assay streptolysin O is the antigen. The activity of this antigen as seen in the assay is

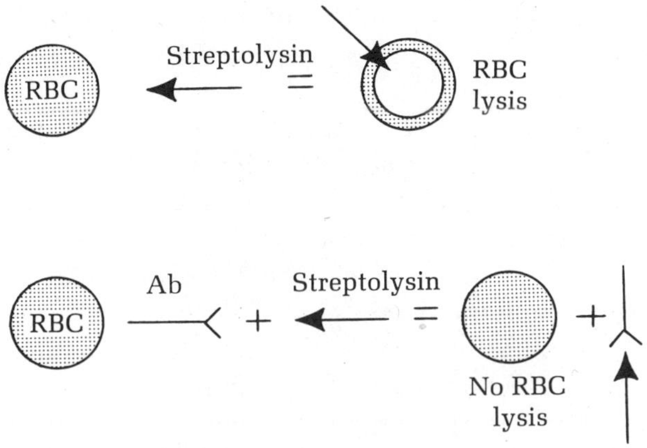

Fig. 8-3. Illustration of anti-streptolysin O reaction. Top demonstrates lytic activity of streptolysin O with group O human red blood cells; bottom shows inhibition of lytic activity by serum antibody collected after streptococcal infection.

red blood cell lysis. As shown in Fig. 8-3, human group O red blood cells readily lyse in the presence of streptolysin O. The hemolytic ability of streptolysin O is inhibited by the neutralizing antibody found in the patient's serum after infection.

Methodology. A variety of specified patient serum dilutions are employed as described by Rantz and Randal. A constant amount of a standardized preparation of streptolysin O is added to dilutions of patient serum and to the reference control. The tests are incubated and then human group O red blood cells are added to each tube. The tests are again incubated. After the second incubation, the tubes are inspected for hemolysis. If a sufficient amount of ASO is present, it will neutralize all streptolysin O in the tube, hence, no hemolysis.

Interpretation. The end point of the ASO is reported in Todd units. Todd units are calculated by taking the reciprocal of the highest dilution that shows no hemolysis. While the assay is very reproducible, it does have some major difficulties. Streptolysin O is relatively labile, and false neutralization of the lytic activity may be interpreted as positive results. Certain bacterial products and beta lipoproteins are capable of neutralizing streptolysin O, resulting in false positive results. Twofold dilution change in titer between acute and convalescent specimens is considered significant and indicates recent group A streptococcal infection. Early treatment with antibiotics and the slow progress of glomerulonephritis usually make it impossible to obtain the recommended paired, acute, and convalescent specimens. For this reason an "upper limit" of normal value is usually used. This upper limit value is age, season, and geographically dependent, but this upper limit is normally considered to be approximately 166 Todd units. Unfortunately, the antibody response to streptolysin O in patients with skin infections caused by streptococci is poor and therefore the diagnostic value, for these patients, in glomerulonephritis is low. Antihyaluronidase or antiDNase-B would be of more value to the clinician when the patient has had skin streptococci infections.

Several controls must be included with each ASO test batch. A reference control is needed to validate (1) the potency of streptolysin O, (2) the technical skills of the personnel, and (3) the quality of the other reagents. A variation of one dilution from the expected value is not acceptable. A streptolysin O red blood cell control monitors the cell suspension and potency of streptolysin O. Clearly this last control should not be hemolyzed.

Elevation of ASO occurs 1 to 3 weeks after infection. The titer normally drops by 8 to 10 weeks after infection. Extremely high titers are most commonly associated with glomerulonephritis and rheumatic fever. High titers are rarely found in other disorders, including pneumonia and other types of streptococcal infections.

READINGS AND RESOURCES

Bennett, C. W.: Clinical serology, Springfield, Ill., 1972, Charles C Thomas, Publisher.

Bidwell, E.: Acquired inhibitors of coagulation, Annu. Rev. Med. **20:**63, 1969.

Cinader, B., editor: Antibodies to biologically active molecules, New York, 1967, Pergamon Press, Inc.

Feinstein, D. I., and Rapaport, S. I.: Acquired inhibitors of blood coagulation, Haemostasis **1:**75, 1972.

Hallen, J.: Non-specific streptolysin O inhibition in diseases of the liver and biliary system, Acta. Pathol. Microbiol. Scand. **57:**301, 1963.

Hierholzer, J. C., Suggs, M. T., and Hall, E. C.: Standardized viral hemagglutination and hemagglutination-inhibition test II. Description and statistical evaluation, Appl. Microbiol. **18:**824, 1969.

Kaplan, E. J., Anthony, B. F., Chapman, S. S., Ayoub, E. M., and Wannamaker, L. W.: The influence of the site of infection on the immune response to group A streptococci, J. Clin. Invest. **49:**1405, 1970.

Kibrick, S., Belding, D. L., and Merrill, B.: Methods for the detection of antibodies against mammalian spermatozoa, II. A gelatin agglutination test, Fertil. Steril. **3:**430, 1952.

Lechner, K.: Acquired inhibitors in non-hemophiliac patients, Haemostasis **3:**65, 1974.

Liao, S. J.: A modification of the antistreptolysin-O test, J. Lab. Clin. Med. **38:**648, 1951.

Miale, J.: Laboratory medicine: hematology, ed. 5, St. Louis, 1977, The C. V. Mosby Co.

Rantz, L. A., and Randall, E.: A modification of the technique for determination of streptolysin-O titer, Proc. Soc. Exp. Biol. Med. **59:**22, 1945.

Rose, N. R., and Friedman, H., editors: Manual of clinical immunology, Washington, D.C., 1976, American Society of Microbiology.

Rose, N. R., Hjort, T., Rumke, M. P., Harper, M., and Vyzaor, O.: Workshop on techniques for the detection of ISO and auto-antibodies to human spermatozoa, Clin. Exp. Immunol. **23:**175, 1976.

Sell, S.: Immunology, immunopathology and immunity, Baltimore, 1972, Harper & Row, Publishers.

CHAPTER 9

Labeled immunoassays

Immunoassays utilize antibody to detect antigen or antigen to detect antibody. These tests show remarkable sensitivity and specificity as compared with other types of chemical reactions. Recently, modifications of the basic principles of immunochemistry are greatly expanding the potential usefulness of these tests. The primary difference between these newer procedures and the previously discussed assays is that the procedures employ labeled or tagged antigen or antibody. The tag is an active molecule that is covalently bound to noncritical free amino or carboxyl groups or is added by other means to the molecule. What advantage does this offer? The tag, owing to its activity, amplifies the power of the test or increases its sensitivity as can be seen through the following analogy. Assume that you were assigned the job of counting skyrockets on the fourth of July. Imagine the difference in trying to count those that were a mere flash of light as compared to those with multiple pyrotechnical displays. The multiple explosive displays are analogous to the tags used in these immunoassays. The displays are active and are readily detectable or visible and make it possible to identify the skyrocket in the night sky. In a similar manner the active molecules bound to antigen or antibody make it possible to observe the antigen-antibody reaction. Generally, the higher the activity of the tag, the more readily we can detect the reaction. The immunoassay becomes more sensitive, reliable, and by far more versatile.

In both research and clinical medicine the types of labeled immunoassays and their applications are proceeding through an enormous growth period. Clinically, these assays are looked at as the ultimate methodologies and they provide the laboratory with powerful tools of extreme sensitivity and specificity. It is reported that some of these procedures are able to detect antigen in concentrations down to 10^{-17} M. Broadly speaking, we can divide these assays into two types, immunomicroscopic and those assays based on competitor receptor binding.

IMMUNOMICROSCOPY

Principles and limitations

In immunomicroscopy one utilizes tagged antibody or antigen to visualize the immune partner. Frequently the antigen is cellular or subcellular and the search is accomplished via the tagged antibody. The label commonly employed may be one of several types including metalloproteins, fluorescein dyes, enzymes, or radioactive isotopes. These labels all have one property in common. This property is that they all have a unique characteristic that, under special circumstances, makes them visible. An antibody tagged with one of these substances in a way holds a flag. When this antibody reacts with an antigen, the location of the flag indicates the site of the antibody, hence the antigen. For example, it is extremely difficult to search for the tuberculosis bacillus in body samples; however, by using labeled antituberculosis antiserum, this task is made easier.

Direct assay. There are two major types of immunomicroscopic techniques. The first technique is the direct method and, as shown in Fig. 9-1, employs fluorescent-labeled antibody and a specially modified light microscope. The direct method uses but a single major reagent; labeled antibody directed at the antigen under investigation. For example, in Fig. 9-1, we could be screening body samples microscopically for the presence of streptococcus organisms. In this case the direct assay would use fluorescent-labeled antistreptococcal antiserum. The microscopic visualization of the label would indicate the presence of the organism. Clearly the assay combines the specificity of the immune reaction with the sensitivity of active labels. Direct assays can be used to detect the presence of a variety of organisms, surface markers on B and T lymphocytes, and so on.

Indirect assay. The indirect techniques are more versatile and less expensive. These tests employ an additional reagent. There are basically three reactants: antigen, specific homologous antibody, and labeled antiantibody. These assays are presently most often used to detect autoantibodies in patient samples; however, with minor modifications in technique they can be used for a wide variety of purposes. In Fig. 9-2, a typical reaction is depicted. Patient serum is allowed to react with an antigen substrate. Unfixed excess serum is carefully washed away with buffer. In the second major step labeled antiserum is used to detect fixed antibody. The labeled antiglobulin will not react with the antigen substrate, for its specificity is toward antibody. A variety of substrates are used in immunomicroscopy, depending on the objective of the assay. The following is a partial list of substrates used in immunomicroscopy.

Autoantibody detection
1. Animal organs, tissues, or cells
2. Human organs, tissues, or cells

Immune complex disease
1. Biopsy of tissue involved

Antibodies to microorganisms
1. Slide-mounted organisms

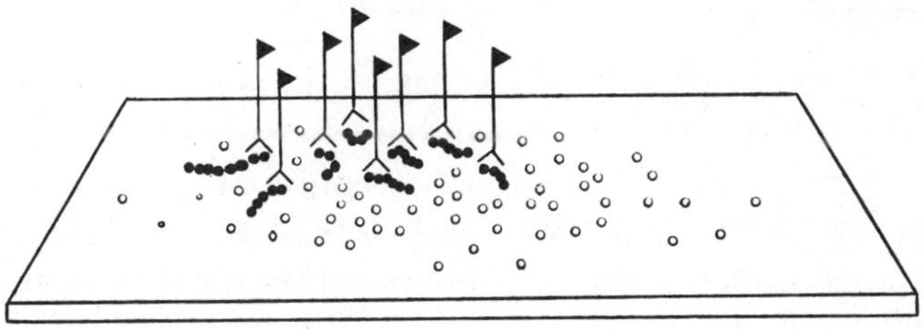

Fig. 9-1. Direct immunomicroscopy. Antibody labeled with flag seeks out and identifies location of difficult to find antigens. Flag is symbol of active molecules; its location indicates presence of antibody reacted with antigen.

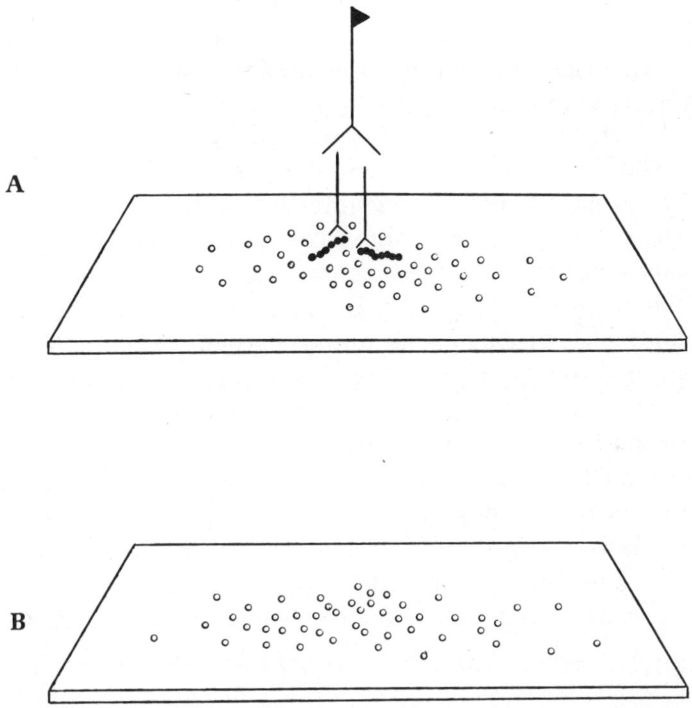

Fig. 9-2. Indirect immunomicroscopy. **A,** Positive reaction. Note that antibody that bears label (flag) is antiglobulin and reaction seems to identify antibody in patient serum. **B,** Assay using patient whose serum contains no antibody to antigen substrate (negative reaction).

Cellular localization of immunoglobulins

1. Bone marrow
2. Lymph nodes
3. Peripheral blood

Localization of microorganism

1. Body fluids and tissues
2. Tissue culture

Fluorescent techniques

Principles. Fluorescent substances have a unique physiochemical property. This unique characteristic is that when these substances absorb light in the ultraviolet light region (200 to 400 nm), they emit a characteristic wavelength of light in the visible region. The wavelength of light emitted and absorbed is specific for each fluor. Using a series of filters within a modified microscope, it is possible to view the light emitted by the fluor against a black background. Using a few mild chemical reactions, it is possible to conjugate one of these fluorescent substances to free amino, carboxyl, or sulfhydryl groups on the antibody molecule (Fig. 9-3). The popularly used fluors include fluorescein, lissamine, rhodamine B, and 1-dimethylaminonapthalene-5 sulfonic acid (DANSYL). The choice of fluor depends on several factors such as the color of autofluorescence of certain tissues. This discussion will be limited to the use of fluorescein isothiocyanate; however, most principles apply to other fluorescent conjugates.

Preparation of fluorescein conjugate. Fluorescein isothiocyanate–labeled (FITC) antibodies are probably the most frequently utilized system in immunomicroscopy. To prepare this labeled conjugate one must begin with a high titer antiserum. The gamma fraction of this antiserum is then purified by a combination of methods, for example, salt precipitation and column fractionation. FITC is chemically combined with the purified antiserum (Fig. 9-3). FITC conjugates to amino or sulfhydryl groups in the antibody protein. FITC will also label other serum protein more readily than immunoglobulins; hence, it is critically important to be dealing with purified immunoglobulins. The major sources of error in preparation of the FITC conjugate are as follows: excessive FITC labeling may lead to nonspecific fluorescence, and harsh handling in purification and labeling may result in loss of antibody activity. After completion of labeling, unbound FITC can be removed by gel filtration. The ratio of FITC to protein (F/P) is very important and is a useful tool in monitoring excessive FITC labeling. The higher the F/P ratio the more electronegative the resulting conjugate. A highly nega-

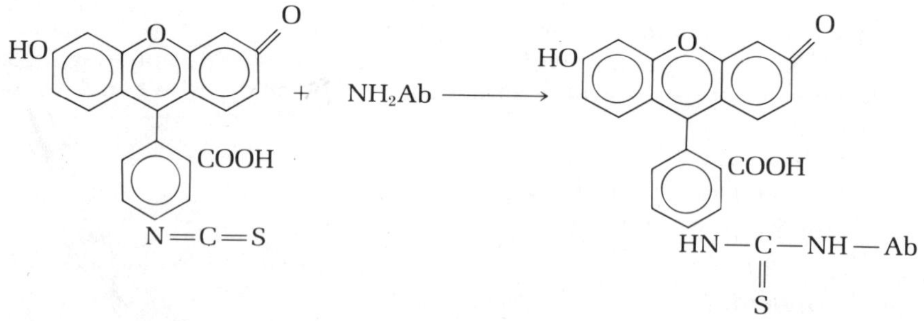

Fig. 9-3. Conjugation of fluor to antibody molecule. Fluorescein isothiocyanate reacts with free amino groups on antibody molecule, resulting in conjugation of fluorescent substance to antibody.

tively charged conjugate will have a greater probability of nonspecific binding to antigen substrate. The molar F/P ratios usually range from 1 to 3 and may be as high as 6 in some assay systems. The titer of antiserum prior to and after conjugation must be monitored for loss of activity. One of the simpler techniques to titer the antiserum is by means of reverse radial diffusion. In the reverse radial diffusion method, antigen is incorporated into the gel while the antiserum diffuses radially from precut wells. The titer is indicated by the highest dilution of antibody that visibly reacts with the antigen-gel combination when the antigen concentration in gel is fixed at 1 mg/ml.

Staining procedure. The labeled antiserum is overlaid on the antigen substrate under investigation. If homologous antigen is present in the substrate, the labeled antibody is fixed. After gentle washing to remove unfixed FITC, the substrate is viewed under a fluorescent microscope. The bound FITC is readily visible as green fluorescent areas against a black background. Variations in the procedure include the indirect assay discussed earlier as well as other modifications.

Quality control. The most useful control methods are accomplished merely by assaying a positive and negative sample with each test. One should be aware that blocking antibody present in the patient sample can mask all homologous antigenic sites and inhibit binding of the FITC conjugate in direct assays. The fluorescent assays are relatively inexpensive, rapid, sensitive, and specific techniques. They are extremely valuable in screening patient samples for autoantibodies. The major disadvantage in fluorescent studies is the high initial investment and the need for skilled personnel. The availability of preconjugated antisera has greatly improved the quality and usefulness of fluorescent study.

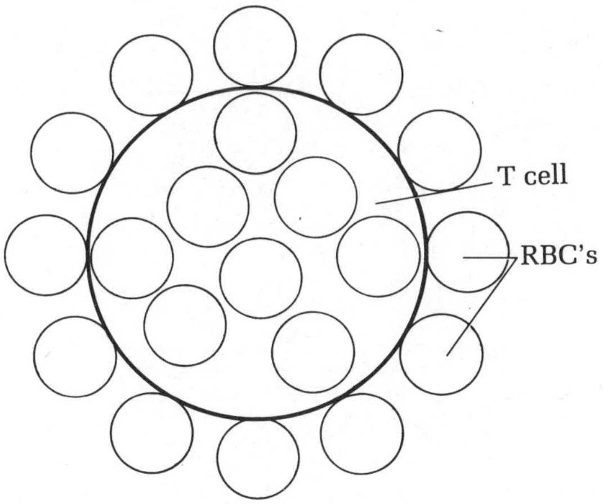

Fig. 9-4. T cell rosette. Sheep red blood cells adhere to surface of T cells forming rosettes; however, mechanism is "nonimmune."

Clinical examples

Lymphocyte surface markers—enumeration of B cells

Principles. The two major groups of lymphocytes, B and T cells, have distinguishable surface structures. The B cell surface is coated with membrane-bound immunoglobulin (mIg). Also present on the B cell surface are receptors for the Fc portion of immunoglobulins and receptors for complement. Approximately 1% to 15% of the peripheral lymphocytes are composed of B cells. This discussion will be limited to two techniques, one to identify the Fc receptor and the other to identify mIg. Both procedures are valuable in enumerating B cells.

Fc receptors. The B cell Fc receptors can be readily estimated through immune rosette formation. If antibody-coated erythrocytes are mixed with a purified lymphocyte preparation, the Fc receptors on B cells will bind antibody yielding rosettes (Fig. 9-5).

A fluorescent technique to visualize the Fc receptors employs labeled immune complexes. The Fc of the labeled antibody within the immune complex binds to the receptors and is visible under the fluorescent microscope. Another technique utilizes pepsin-digested IgG. Pepsin cleaves IgG heavy chains in the hinge region and one of the products is the Fc fragment. This Fc fragment can then be labeled and used to identify Fc receptors.

Surface immunoglobulins (mIg). Conjugated antisera specific for IgM and IgG are usually used in a fluorescent assay for mIg (membrane immunoglobulin). The majority of detectable surface immunoglobulin is of the IgM and IgG class.

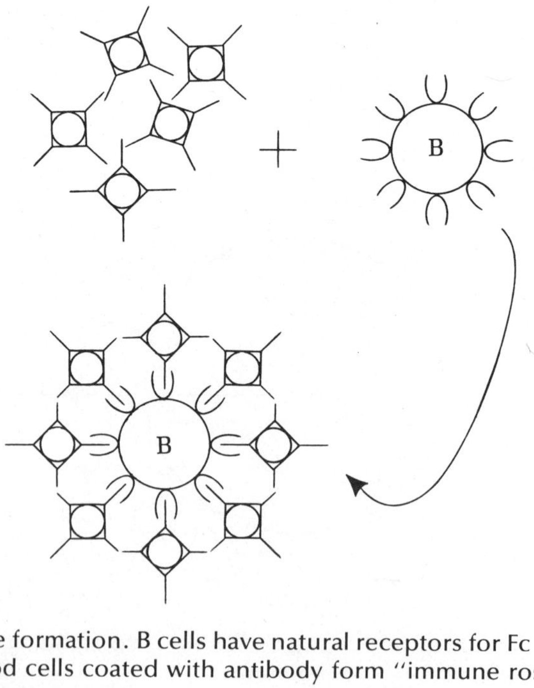

Fig. 9-5. B cell rosette formation. B cells have natural receptors for Fc region of antibody molecules. Red blood cells coated with antibody form "immune rosettes."

Procedure. Mononuclear cells are separated from peripheral blood or bone marrow via Ficoll-Hypaque centrifugation. Since monocytes may be confused with B cells, it is necessary to brand the monocytes with some distinguishing and easily recognized mark. This can be accomplished by incubating the mononuclear cell preparation with latex particles. During incubation these phagocytic cells will engulf the particles, and later the particles can be seen microscopically within the monocytes. The cell suspension is washed thoroughly with buffered saline solution. After washing a mixture of equal volumes of cell suspension and conjugated antiserum, the mixture is incubated in plastic tubes for 30 minutes at room temperature. The suspension is washed several times with buffered saline solution to remove unbound conjugate, then it is centrifuged into a tight pellet. The pellet of cells is resuspended in a drop of buffered saline solution and placed on a glass slide. The suspension is viewed under a fluorescent microscope and the (1) nonfluorescent cells, (2) fluorescent cells, and (3) fluorescent cells with latex inclusions are enumerated.

Interpretation. The value of B and T cell estimates is only recently being appreciated and is still considered somewhat of a research technique. An increase in one particular type of cell adds evidence to the possibility of malignancy. An increased percentage of B lymphocytes is associated with a variety of lymphoproliferative malignancies. Following is a list of lymphoproliferative disorders associated with increased B cell numbers.

1. Acute lymphocytic leukemia
2. Chromic lymphocytic leukemia
3. Waldenströms macroglobulinemia
4. Multiple myeloma

The second major group of patients in which diagnoses are aided includes those with primary immunodeficiencies as shown in Table 21. These patients are highly susceptible to recurring infections. Once a diagnosis is made, the therapeutic response may also be evaluated by monitoring changes in percentages of cell types. Major sources of error in cell enumeration are frequently encountered. As mentioned, one difficulty arises in distinguishing monocytes and lymphocytes. This source of error may be substantial in patients who exhibit

Table 21. Primary immunodeficiency with associated cellular defect

Deficiency	Cellular defect
X-linked agammaglobulinemia	B
Thymic hypoplasia	T
Combined immunodeficiency	B, T
IgA deficiency	B
Ataxia-telangiectasia	B, T
Wiskott-Aldrich syndrome	T
Transient hypoglobulinemia (infantile)	B

monocytosis, for example, certain malignancies, chronic infections and so on. Some patients such as those with systemic lupus erythematosus (SLE) have autoantibodies directed at their own lymphocytes. These patients may then have T cells with what appears to be surface immunoglobulin. Antilymphocyte antibodies are also found in patients with other autoimmune disorders as well as occasionally in infectious mononucleosis. It is likely that, as the popularity of these techniques for B and T cell enumeration increases, medicine will gain new insight into pathologic mechanisms and therapeutic successes.

Antinuclear antibodies

Principles. In a variety of states, including autoimmune disorders, infectious diseases, and normally in aging, the individual may build an immune response to nuclear components. Some of the nuclear components that may react antigenically are double-stranded DNA, single-stranded DNA, histones, basic nucleoproteins, Smith antigen (extractable nuclear antigen), complex ribonucleoprotein, and nucleolar RNA. Immunomicroscopy is an extremely useful tool for evaluating serum for this group of autoantibodies. Using an indirect fluorescent technique a cellular substrate such as rat liver is flooded with patient sample. The patient's antinuclear antibody, if present, binds with nuclear antigens. After incubation and thorough washing with phosphate-buffered saline (PBS) solution, the slide is flooded with fluorescein-conjugated antihuman serum. The slide is again thoroughly washed to remove unbound FITC conjugate and then observed under a fluorescent microscope for nuclear staining patterns. Almost any tissue may be used, but rat liver, kidney, or stomach are the tissues of choice.

Procedure. Patient serum and controls are diluted 1 : 20 with buffered saline solution. This dilution may be used to screen all patients. All assays that are positive when diluted 1 : 20 are then further titrated and the straining pattern is carefully described. The cryostat-cut substrates are mounted on etched slides and kept frozen at −20° C. A separate substrate is used for each sample and the slides are labeled appropriately. A simplified scheme is shown in the boxed material. The pattern of staining is usually described as rim, solid, homogeneous, speckled, or nucleolar in character.

Interpretation. A variety of conditions are known to be associated with positive antinuclear antibody (ANA) reactions, including SLE, scleroderma, dermatomyositis, rheumatoid arthritis, other collagen diseases, malignancies, and hypersensitivity states. Positive ANA reactions occur in low titers in various viral diseases, chronic hepatitis, and frequently in aging. Low titer positive reactions are highly sensitive but poorly specific. As the titer increases so does the specificity of the assay. The greatest diagnostic value in ANA testing is in attempting to rule out SLE in a patient with a complicated clinical picture. Approximately 99% of the patients with active SLE will demonstrate markedly elevated ANA titers. The assay also has some value in monitoring the therapeutic effect of various medications, since generally effective treatment results in a fall in the ANA titer. Anti-DNA, although far less sensitive than the ANA, is considered highly specific

Schematic fluorescein antinuclear antibody (ANA) procedure*

Label slides with diamond pencil
↓
Make 1 : 20 dilution of samples with PBS (or titer)
↓
Apply sample dilution or control to substrate slides
↓
Incubate, moist ambient temperature, for 30 minutes
↓
Decant samples and PBS rinse
↓
Shake off excess PBS
↓
Apply FITC anti-IgG to slides
↓
Incubate, ambient temperature, for 30 minutes
↓
Decant antiserum, rinse in PBS
↓
Wash 10 minutes in PBS with agitation
↓
Air dry
↓
Cover slip mount
↓
Examine for fluorescent apple-green staining

*Modification of Bioware ANA scheme, Bioware, Inc. Wichita, Kansas.

for SLE, especially when combined with C3 and C4 analysis. Anti-DNA can be evaluated via radioimmunoassay (Farr technique).

Enzyme techniques

Principles and limitations. Horseradish peroxidase is an enzyme with a molecular weight of 40,000 daltons. This enzyme is capable of freeing oxygen from hydrogen peroxide (H_2O_2). By coupling these reagents with an oxidizable dye, it is possible to free oxygen and utilize the freed oxygen to cause a color change in the dye. In the peroxidase ANA, the principle just mentioned is utilized in a modification of the fluorescent procedures, which can be read with a light microscope. In this enzyme immunoassay, the enzyme is conjugated, as FITC was, to the antibody molecule. This enzyme can be detected several ways but the most common is histochemical and is based on the reaction shown in Fig. 9-6. The stain utilized is DAB-HCL (3,3-diaminobenzidine hydrochloride), which

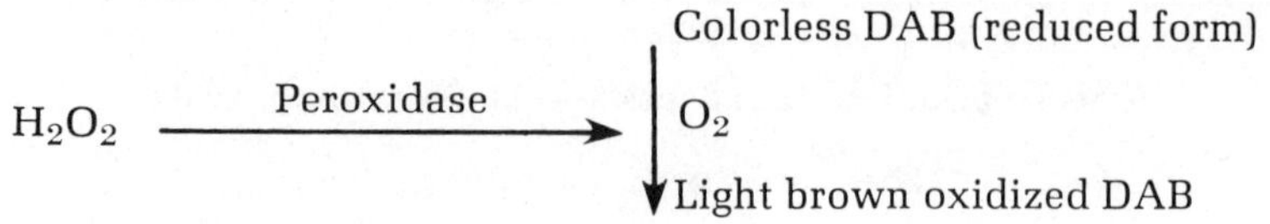

Fig. 9-6. DAB reaction when oxidized in peroxidase antinuclear reaction.

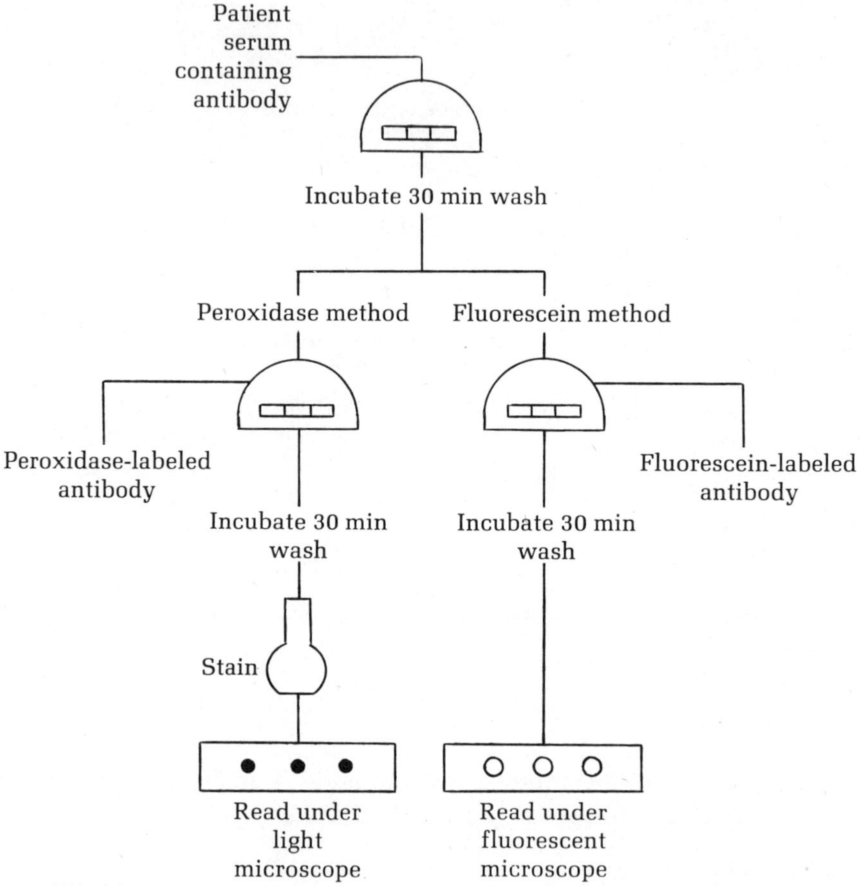

Fig. 9-7. Comparison of techniques used in indirect immunomicroscopy, fluorescent versus peroxidase. (Reproduced with the permission of L. P. Cawley, M.D. and Barbara Minard.)

is colorless in the reduced form and light brown in the oxidized form. The reagents employed are substrate slides, patient serum or controls, peroxidase-labeled anti-IgG, and DAB-HCL with H_2O_2. A comparison of the procedure for peroxidase antinuclear antibody and FITC antinuclear antibody is shown in Fig. 9-7. As can be seen, there are a great many similarities in technique.

Certain problems do exist with the peroxidase ANA procedure. If antibody is excessively burdened with peroxidase label, nonspecific staining may occur. Nonspecific staining may also occur owing to excessive concentration of H_2O_2. Many factors and substances may liberate oxygen from hydrogen peroxide including strong light. A wide variety of substances, in theory, may oxidize DAB-HCL. However, careful preparation and adherence to the described procedure result in data that are comparable to the FITC antinuclear antibody. The major advantage to this technique is that it requires no initial major expense for a fluorescent microscope while maintaining the capability to perform assays that are comparable to those done with fluorescent systems. A broad selection of peroxidase and fluorescent-conjugated antisera is commercially available (Bioware Inc. Wichita, Kansas). By changing substrates it is possible to detect a number of other types of autoantibodies with the same procedures just discussed. It is possible to detect antibodies to mitochondria, smooth muscle, parietal cells, striated muscle, thyroid tissue, myelin, cardiac tissue, skin, colon, glomerulus, and so on.

COMPETITIVE RECEPTOR ASSAYS

Principles and limitations

Competitive receptor assays are a group of tests that have been, and will likely continue to be, extremely beneficial to clinical laboratory medicine. Some people consider this technique as important a development as the development of spectrophotometry. The competitive assays are extremely sensitive, with reports of sensitivity as low as 1×10^{-17} M. While exhibiting this high sensitivity, the assays are extremely versatile. The labels employed are active molecules, and the degree of activity in these labels is one factor that is directly related to assay sensitivity.

The principle of these sophisticated assays is not complex. The substance under investigation in the patient sample competes for binding sites with a similar substance that is labeled. The higher the concentration of this substance in the patient sample, the greater the probability of displacing the labeled form from the available binding sites (Fig. 9-8). The receptors employed in these assays range from cellular binding sites and binding proteins to specific antisera.

In the competitive immunoreceptor assays labeled antigen and homologous antigen (or hapten and homologous hapten) in the patient sample compete for Fab sites on the antiserum. To quantitate the displacement one may measure the free form of the labeled antigen that is directly related to the patient antigen concentration or the bound form. The bound-labeled antigen activity is inversely related to the concentration of homologous antigen in the patient sample. Note equations 9-1 and 9-2, which demonstrate the reaction of antigen and antibody in these assays. When the labeled antigen (Ag^*) is allowed to react with limited binding sites, free and bound label is distributed as follows:

$$12\ Ag^* + 6\ Ab \rightleftharpoons 6\ Ag^*Ab + 6\ Ag^* \qquad \textbf{(Eq. 9-1)}$$

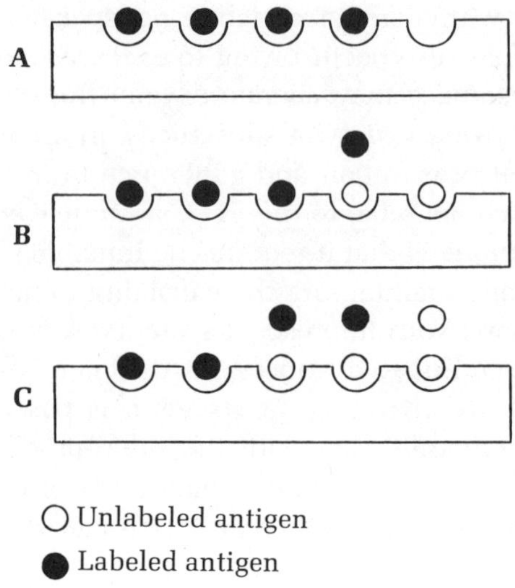

Fig. 9-8. Receptor-binding assays. Note that labeled antigen bound to receptor sites is displaced by homologous antigen present in patient's sample. **A,** Patient sample is free of substance understudy. **B** and **C,** Increasing concentrations of homologous antigen in patient samples.

When patient sample, control, or standards contain homologous-labeled antigen, displacement of the labeled Ag occurs.

$$12\ Ag^* + 6\ Ab + 6\ Ag \rightleftharpoons 2\ Ag^*Ab + 4\ AgAb + 10\ Ag^* + 2\ Ag \qquad \textbf{(Eq. 9-2)}$$

Note the increased free-labeled antigen and the decreased bound-labeled antigen. Labels currently used in these receptor assays include radioactive isotopes, enzymes, and electron spin radicals. The techniques are called by various names depending on the labeling and receptor systems, for example, competitive protein binding, radioligand binding, radioimmunoassay, saturation analysis, displacement analysis, enzyme immunoassay, and spin immunoassays.

Radioimmunoassay

Principle and applications. Much of the credit for the present success of radioimmunoassay (RIA) should be given to Berson and Yalow. In the late 1950's they performed a monumental series of experiments that have endowed clinical medicine and research with this powerful analytical tool. In their initial work they injected two groups of patients with ^{131}I-labeled insulin. One group had never received insulin while the other group was composed of diabetics who frequently received insulin. They observed that the diabetics cleared the labeled insulin slower than the nondiabetic group. Electrophoretic fractioning of the diabetics' serum was done, and it was found that the ^{131}I was in a gamma globulin region. The diabetics had developed insulin antibodies that bound the injected insulin. Recognizing the need for an accurate, sensitive assay for plasma insulin, they proceeded to develop the first RIA. Since that time, the basic concepts generated by Berson and Yalow's work have been utilized in a vast number of assays as shown in the following boxed material.

A partial listing of commercially available radioimmunoassay test kits

Nonpeptide hormones	Peptide hormones
Cortisone	Growth hormone
Aldosterone	Adrenocortical hormone
Testosterone	Thyrotropin-releasing factor
Estrogen	Human chorionic gonadotropin
Nonhormonal substances	
Digitoxin	Thyroid-binding globulin
Digoxin	Australian antigen
Dilantin	IgE
Morphine	C-reactive protein
Carcinoembryonic antigen	
Alpha-fetoprotein	

Radioimmunoassay has been shown to combine the specificity of the immune reaction with the sensitivity of high specific-activity isotopes. The basic procedure used in RIA is similar to that of other competitive binding assays. In separate tubes a constant amount of antisera is mixed with a constant amount of labeled antigen. To each of these tubes either patient sample, control, or one of several standards are added. During incubation homologous unlabeled antigen tends to displace labeled antigen from binding sites as is exemplified in equations 9-1 and 9-2. Once an equilibrium is reached, the next critical step is to determine the radioactivity of the free antigen, bound antigen, or both the free and bound antigen fractions. Since the radioactivity is equally measurable in both fractions, it is necessary to rapidly and completely separate free antigen from bound antigen. A number of techniques are available to accomplish rapid separation; some of these will be discussed. Once separated it is necessary to determine the radioactive decay rate of the free or bound fraction (sometimes both are determined). The method of determining radioactivity depends on the available instrumentation, the number of assays, and the isotope used. A calibration curve or dose-reponse curve is generated by plotting a parameter of radioactivity versus antigen concentration. This curve can utilize the decay rate (counts per minute) of the bound fraction, the percent bound, the ratio of bound over free, or the free fraction. The dose-response curve shown in Fig. 9-9 plots the concentration of

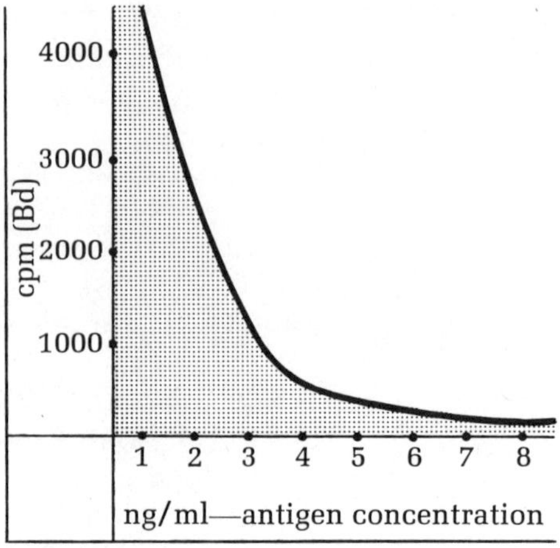

Fig. 9-9. Dose-response curve or calibration curve plotting decay in bound (Bd) fraction versus antigen concentration in nanograms per milliliter. Typically used calibration curve for radioimmunoassay.

Table 22. Comparative characteristics of isotopes used in RIA

Isotope	Half-life	Specific activity (approx.)	Emission
^{131}I	8 days	10^6 cpm/ng	Gamma
^{125}I	57 days	10^5 cpm/ng	Gamma
^{3}H	12 years	10^3 cpm/ng	Beta
^{14}C	5600 years	10^1 cpm/ng	Beta

each standard versus the activity (cpm) of the bound fraction. From this curve the patient antigen levels can readily be interpolated.

Purification of antigen. The specificity of the antiserum used in the assay is obviously important. One can improve the quality of an antiserum through various procedures such as absorption. However, the best way to assure the quality of the antiserum is through the use of a purified antigen when eliciting the antiserum. Prior to immunization of the animal the antigen is purified using several separation techniques, some of which were discussed in Chapter 1, for example, gel and ion exchange chromatography. After completion of purification, part of the antigen is used to elicit an antibody response and part is labeled and used in the assay as homologous antigen.

Labeling of antigen. A primary concern in antigen labeling is choice of isotope. Before proceeding one must consider the specific activity of radionuclides. Specific activity expresses the activity per unit quantity of the isotope sample. Several units may be used to express specific activity such as decays per minute per m mole. The sensitivity of the assay is highly dependent on specific activity.

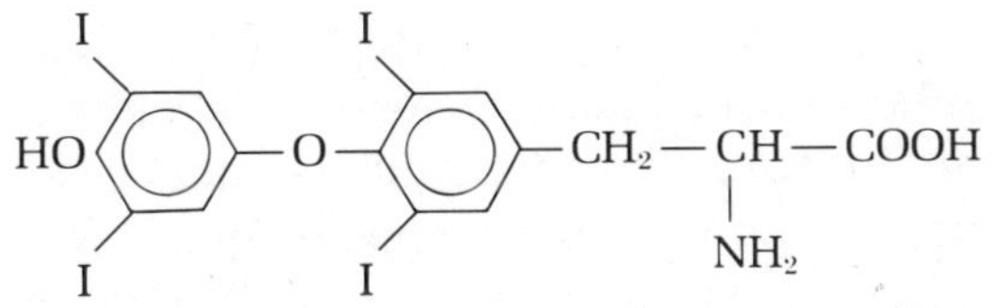

Fig. 9-10. Thyroxine structure. Note iodine positions that are natural sites for substitution with radioactive isotopes of iodine.

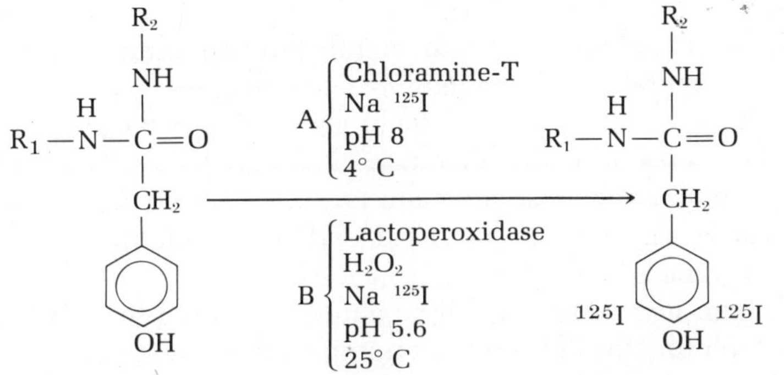

Fig. 9-11. Two unnatural methods for addition of radioactive iodine. Note tyrosine is necessary receptor in both.

Low specific-activity isotopes require the use of greater amounts of isotope and result in loss of sensitivity. An assay that employs a label decaying at a rate of 10^6 dpm/ng will be easier to detect than one that is decaying at a rate of 10^3 dpm/ng.

Some substances naturally contain elements that have radioactive isotopes. Owing to the dynamic state of molecules, these substances will readily exchange nonradioactive elements for radioactive isotopes. This is easily acomplished with ^{3}H or ^{14}C, since most molecules contain carbon and hydrogen atoms. Molecules that have iodine within the structure will readily exchange ^{131}I or ^{125}I for elemental iodine. A good example of this is thyroxine, shown in Fig. 9-10. The high specific activity of ^{131}I and ^{125}I has promoted their use in RIA. Most clinical laboratories have utilized gamma-emitting isotopes for decades and therefore are aware of the proper care and handling. These laboratories are already equipped with the necessary instrumentation capable of counting the gamma emissions of ^{125}I with greater efficiency than the emissions of ^{131}I. When comparing ^{131}I to ^{125}I, it would appear that the shorter half-life of ^{131}I would favor its usage. However, a short half-life has a disadvantage, for in 2 weeks ^{131}I looses 75% of its activity.

The increased interest in the use of ^{125}I for antigen labeling in RIA has created several problems. Most antigens do not contain iodine; hence substitution is impossible. It is possible, with certain chemical and enzymatic reactions, to iodinate noniodine-containing molecules as shown in Fig. 9-11.

Although increased activity of the isotope tends to increase the sensitivity of the assay, there are other considerations. Excessive labeling may cause radiation damage to the antigen. In RIA both patient antigen and labeled homologous antigen must be identical in order that they compete equally for binding sites.

Evaluation of antiserum. There are three primary considerations in evaluating an antiserum for use in RIA. The antiserum should have a high titer, good specificity, and reasonable affinity. The antiserum is generally prepared via the classical techniques of immunization discussed in Chapter 3. Small molecules, usually with molecular weights less than 10,000, require conjugation to carrier proteins prior to animal immunization. Highly purified antigens are used in low to moderate concentrations in the immunization process. Current thought suggests that only high-affinity surface immunoglobulins of lymphocytes will bind antigens of low concentrations, therefore eliciting only high-affinity antibody. The last and sometimes a most important factor to consider is luck. An animal's immune response is genetically controlled, and in any immunization effort a certain number of animals just will not respond to a particular antigen. The antiserum must have a high titer so that it can be diluted and used in a large number of assays. When diluting the antiserum, it is important to consider that in any competitive assay there must be a limited number of binding sites. If binding sites were not limited, competition would not be an efficient procedure. The choice of dilution is not a matter of random dilution, rather the dilution used should be one that binds 50% of the labeled antigen in the absence of homologous unlabeled antigen or as shown in Fig. 9-12 when bound fraction (B/F) is equal to one. Overdilution will result in loss of sensitivity in the assay. As shown in Fig. 9-13, only large changes in antigen concentration will displace labeled antigen. The standard curve is an excellent tool to evaluate assay sensitivity. As can be seen

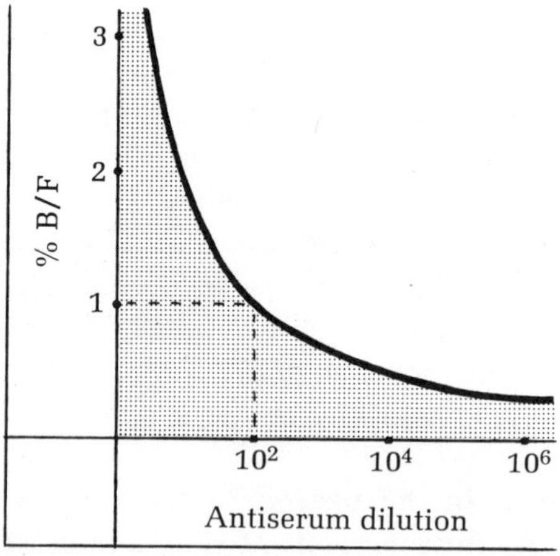

Fig. 9-12. Dose-response curve plotted by using B/F versus dilutions of antiserum with only labeled antigen present, B/F equals one at an antiserum dilution of 10^2.

in Fig. 9-14, changes in the antiserum with time may elaborate varying curves. Curves A, B, and C are different curves obtained with the same kit on different days. On day 1, curve A showed maximum steepness, hence highest sensitivity. On curve A extremely small changes in concentration of unlabeled antigen result in enormous changes in counts per minute in both the bound and free fractions. As time passes, curves B and C have lost much of this sensitivity. Many antisera prepared versus insulin are capable of detecting a single amino acid change between porcine and human insulin. The degree of specificity an antiserum exhibits is a characteristic of each antiserum. Cross-reactivity can be reduced by absorbing the antiserum with carrier molecules and possible cross-reactive substances.

Prior to initiating the use of a new procedure, the selectivity of the immune recognition system should be assessed. The specificity can be checked by screening with similar commonly present substances. The degree of cross-reactivity is closely related to the affinity of the antiserum. While in many respects it is desirable to have a high-affinity antiserum, it holds true that the higher the affinity the more likely binding will occur between antibody and heterologous, structurally similar molecules. On the other side, low-affinity antiserum will not efficiently bind antigen or may reduce the sensitivy of the assay. Unfortunately,

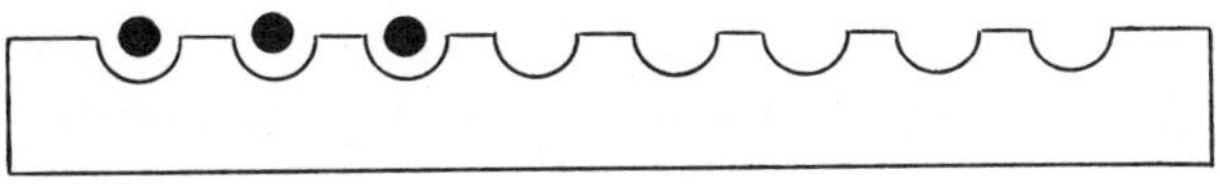

Fig. 9-13. Excess binding sites. At least six unlabeled antigen molecules are necessary to displace single labeled antigen.

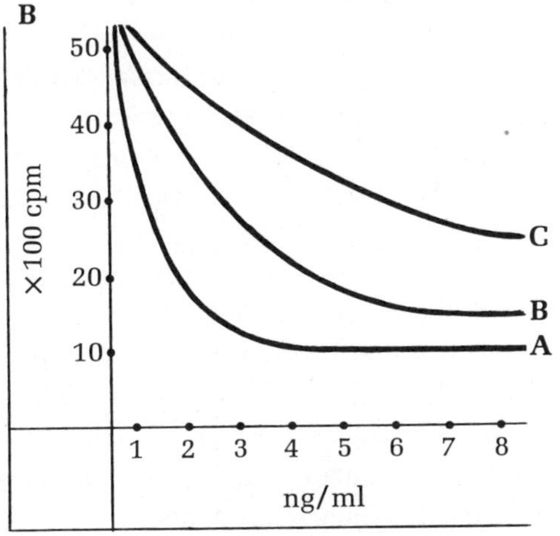

Fig. 9-14. Demonstration of decay of standard curves on 3 days. Note loss of sensitivity with time, curve *A* is on day 1, while curve *B* and *C* are assays on later days.

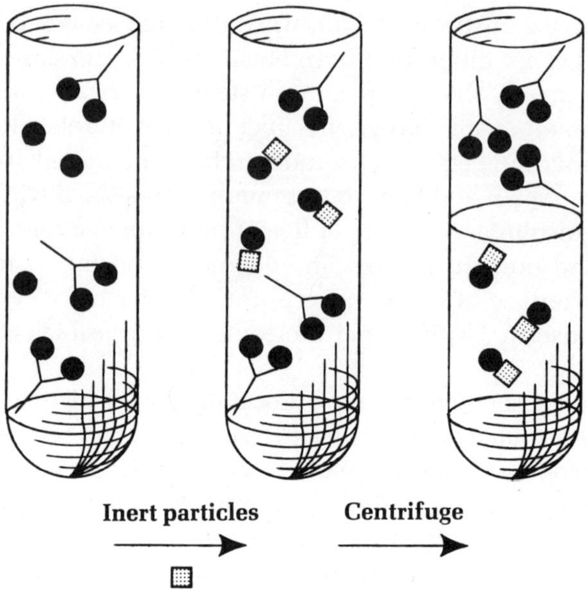

Fig. 9-15. Separation of free antigen from antibody-bound antigen by absorption of free antigen to inert particles. Antigen absorbed to particles is readily separated via centrifugation.

all this highly sophisticated science breaks down at this point to luck and trial and error. Nonspecific interferences of binding occur as discussed in Chapter 4. The most common offenders of antibody-binding interference are pH, hyperbilirubinemia, heparin, or excessively high temperatures.

Separation techniques. As mentioned earilier, rapid separation of free and bound antigen is a critical point in all RIA procedures. Since antibody-bound antigen and free antigen are physically and chemically different, it is possible to bring about separation by a variety of techniques. Antibody-bound antigen is rapidly separated from free antigen by most chromatographic methods, including electrophoresis, ion exchange, or molecular sieving techniques. However, in these techniques timing, pH, and ionic strength are critical and are major sources of error. Absorption of free antigen to inert particles followed by centrifugation is a popular method. Particles such as dextran, talc, or charcoal are frequently utilized in absorption techniques. Absorption separation techniques were the first practical separation methods; however, there are several problems with this method. Problems with timing, suspension uniformity, and protein interference, have caused scientists to seek out more effective techniques. Salt precipitation (Chapter 1) of an RIA mixture will result in precipitation of all globulins. Precipitating globulins is, in reality, separating bound antigen from free antigen, leaving free antigen in solution and bound in the precipitate. Salt or solvent can be used to precipitate globulins and both are inexpensive methods. Unfortunately, these methods are relatively destructive to the immune complex and tend to cause disruption. A certain amount of nonspecific globulin binding tends to occur.

A technique that has gained much popularity is the double antibody procedure. In this elaborate, yet simple, procedure an antiglobulin induced in a different species of animal is used to induce precipitation of the bound antigen, as shown in equations 9-3 and 9-4.

$$\text{Rabbit antidigoxin} + \text{Digoxin} \rightarrow \text{Soluble rabbit anti-Dig-Dig} \qquad \textbf{(Eq. 9-3)}$$

$$\text{Goat antirabbit globulin} + \text{Rabbit anti-Dig-Dig} \rightarrow \text{Precipitation} \qquad \textbf{(Eq. 9-4)}$$

The double antibody technique gives better than a 95% separation of bound and free antigen. It is a highly sensitive technique and not as susceptible to the common sources of error: time, pH, temperature, or other differences in patient samples. The double antibody method is expensive, and the centrifuged immune complex pellet is fragile and easily disrupted. Two methods employing the double antibody technique are frequently used, the post- and pre-precipitate procedures. As can be seen in equation 9-5, the pre-precipitate procedures employ a single double antibody reagent. The pre-precipitate procedures tend to reduce performance time. Equations 9-3 and 9-4 are examples of the post-precipitate procedures.

$$Ab_1\ Ab_2 + Ag \rightarrow Ab_1Ab_2Ag \qquad \textbf{(Eq. 9-5)}$$

A present procedure in vogue utilizes a solid-phase primary antibody. In these techniques the antibodies are linked to particles or to the inside of glass tubes. Solid-phase procedures greatly simplify RIA. All test reactants are added to the solid phase assay tube, incubated, decanted, and washed with buffer. Separation occurs as a result of decanting and washing; bound antigen remains fixed to the solid phase while the free antigen is discarded. Solid-phase procedures produce excellent separation and reduce assay time. The factors that oppose the use of solid-phase techniques are many. They are expensive, less sensitive, and less precise than the classical double antibody procedures.

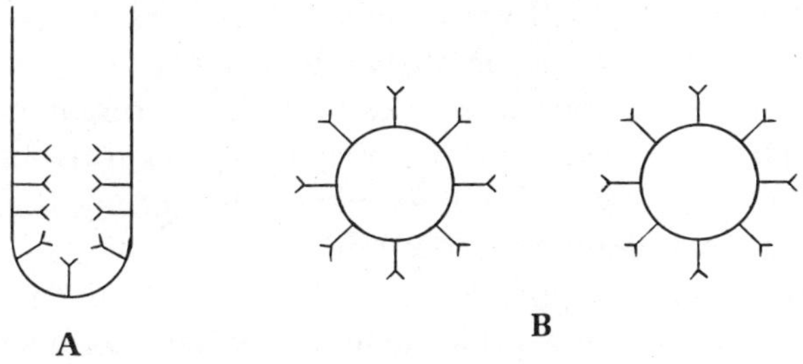

Fig. 9-16. Two solid-phase separation methods that employ antibody covalently bound to solid medium. **A,** Antibody is linked to inner wall of glass test tubes. **B,** Antibody is bound to glass beads.

Standard curves. After separation is complete the next step in all RIA procedures is to generate a dose-response curve, more commonly known as the standard curve. Depending on the procedure or personal preference either the bound, the free, or both fractions are evaluated for radioactivity. The counting technique depends primarily on the type of isotope used as a label (Table 18). Radioactive isotopes that emit gamma rays (^{125}I) are counted in a crystal scintillation counter. The RIA tube containing the bound isotope or the free isotope is lowered into a thallium-doped sodium iodide crystal. The unique feature of this iodide crystal is that when it interacts with gamma rays a short flash of light is released. The crystal is enveloped in foil to protect it from extraneous light. The light flashes are detected by a photomultiplier tube that is sealed to one end of the crystal. The photomultiplier tube detects, converts, and amplifies the light impulses into measurable impulses of electricity, which are then counted.

Beta-emitting isotopes must be evaluated in a different manner. The beta particle is enormous in size compared to the gamma ray. Because of the size of beta particles, they have poor penetration power and are unable to penetrate the glass tube used in the assay. To overcome this problem the selected assay fraction, bound or free, is mixed with a liquid fluor in a procedure known as liquid scintillation. The beta emission interacts with the fluor producing light flashes. The light flashes are picked up by photomultiplier tubes and counted. In a liquid scintillator either beta- or gamma-emitting isotopes may be evaluated. Included in each assay run is a zero standard and five different standard concentrations in duplicate along with paired controls and duplicate samples for each patient. The counts for the zero tube are used when calculating the percent of the total labeled antigen, which is antibody bound, as shown in equation 9-6.

$$\%\ \text{Bd} = \frac{\text{Sample activity} - \text{Background activity}}{\text{Activity in the zero tube} - \text{Background activity}} \qquad \textbf{(Eq. 9-6)}$$

The dose-response curve is then prepared by plotting the percent bound (B/F) or free for each standard versus that standard's concentration. The dose-reponse curve shown in Fig. 9-17, was prepared by plotting the percent bound for each standard versus its concentration. Most curves (Fig. 9-17) are hyperparabolic. The advent of computers in RIA has caused much interest in linearizing the curve. This can sometimes be accomplished by what is called a logit transformation. In the logit transformation one takes logarithmic function of the dose and percent of bound fraction to plot the dose response. Linear regions of the calibration curves can occasionally be obtained merely by plotting decay counts of the bound fraction versus antigen concentration.

Quality control. A high degree of accuracy and precision can be attained with RIA. Several studies have shown that neither precision nor accuracy is affected to any great extent by using beta-emitting labels instead of gamma-emitting labels. Several important pitfalls do exist with RIA. One of the major problems is in relation to the concept itself. All immunoassays measure immunoreactivity

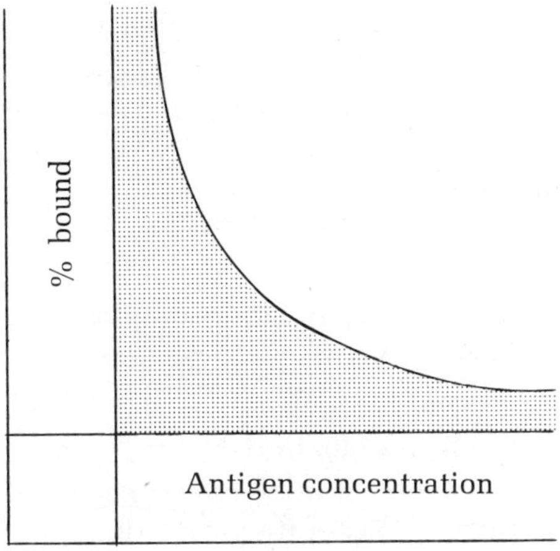

Fig. 9-17. Typical dose-response (calibration) curve for radioimmunoassay.

or antigenicity not biologic activity. Degradation products of hormones or non-active abnormal molecules may be measured in any RIA procedure. Although this is not a problem that can be controlled in the routine RIA laboratory, all people concerned with RIA use must be aware of the problem. At first glance this appears to be a problem without a solution. If the antiserum is prepared against only the active portion of each substance under study, then most of the difficulty is solved. There are at least three major areas that require monitoring when performing RIA:

1. Standard curve data
2. Control sera data
3. Reagent quality and instrumentation

Collection of data on standard curves can be a most fruitful procedure. By comparing each curve with prior curves from a particular RIA kit it is possible to detect losses in sensitivity (note Fig. 9-14). At least two controls should be included with easy assay. These controls should have concentrations that are at medically decisive levels. It is also useful to have the control spiked with potential cross-reactive substances to monitor immune recognition. The data collected with controls should be graphically displayed and statistically analyzed. Reagents, particularly buffers, should be periodically checked for contamination or deterioration. The integrity of the instrumentation is usually checked by counting a known radioactive standard such as cesium and the expected and obtained results should be properly recorded. Proper care of isotopes and use of quality control provide overriding assurance to the analyst and the diagnostician that each assay is valid.

Digoxin

Principles. One of the most extensively used RIA procedures is the quantitative assay for a group of therapeutic compounds known as cardiac glycosides. The

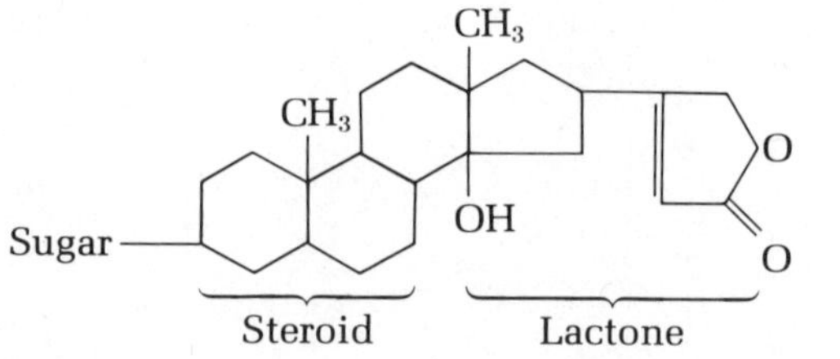

Fig. 9-18. Molecular structure of digoxin and immunodominant steroid nucleus and lactone and sugar side groups.

most popularly used glycoside is digoxin. Digoxin is primarily prescribed for the patient who accumulates excessive fluid, for example, in congestive heart failure. This drug improves the contratibility of the heart, thereby restoring normal circulatory function. The major effects of digoxin therapy include augmented cardiac contractility and irritability, slowing of the heart rate, and slowing of conduction of impulses in the heart muscle. While the cardiac glycoside goup of drugs are important pharmacologic agents, they do have several severe untoward effects. Digoxin side-effects include loss of appetite, nausea, diarrhea, confusion, visual disturbances, and a blocking effect of impulses in cardiac tissue.

Digoxin is eliminated from the body mainly through renal excretion. Elimination through the biliary route is negligible. The diagnosis of digoxin intoxication cannot be made by serum assay alone. However, a knowledge of the digoxin blood level will aid in determining appropriate therapeutic dosages for many patients. Low serum digoxin levels are frequently seen in patients with poor intestinal absorption or those who rapidly metabolize the drug. Low blood levels are often found in the confused, unreliable, or unresponsive patient who cannot be depended on to take medications at the prescribed intervals. Owing to the fact that digoxin is normally excreted via the kidneys, patients with poor renal clearance require a much lower dose to attain therapeutic blood levels. Digoxin retention generally closely parallels the creatinine clearance.

The RIA procedures for digoxin utilize either ^{3}H- or ^{125}I-labeled digoxin. There are both theoretical and real advantages and disadvantages to using one or the other isotope. The ^{125}I procedure invovles the competitive binding of 3-0-succinyl digoxingenin tyrosine ^{125}I with the patient's circulating drug for available binding sites. The steroid nucleus of the digoxin molecule is immunodominant, hence when digoxin, a hapten, is complexed with bovine albumin, immunization results in an antiserum that will likely be suitable for RIA. There are RIA digoxin kits commercially available that employ different separation techniques than ^{125}I or ^{3}H.

Procedure

Solid phase digoxin ^{125}I. Goat antibody to digoxin is covalently coupled to porous glass beads, which in turn are suspended in buffered saline solution. The antibody-coated glass beads are commercially available in prepared tubes (Corning Biological Prod. Dept., Medfield Mass.). Duplicate tubes are labeled with 0, 0.5, 1.0, 2.5, 5,0, and 10.0 ng/ml digoxin. A precise quantity of each standard (200 μl) is added to the appropriate tube; controls and patient samples are pipetted in a similar manner in duplicate tubes. The zero standard is added to the tube marked 0 ng/ml and to tubes marked total counts. Labeled digoxin is added to all tubes. The tubes are then mixed well and incubated so that competition can occur. After 30 minutes the tubes are centrifuged to separate bound isotope from free. Because antibody is immobilized on large inert particles, they are readily sedimented upon centrifugation. Separation is completed by decanting all tubes except the total count tube. All tubes are then assessed for rate of decay via crystal scintillation.

Interpretation. Before elaborating a dose-response curve it is necessary to calculate the percent of the total labeled antigen that is antibody bound, as shown in equation 9-4. Duplicate counts that are greater than 10% apart should be disregarded and repeated. The percent bound for each standard is plotted on semilog paper versus its digoxin concentration. Patient and control results are interpolated from the dose-response curve. It is impossible to predict toxicity from the results of the serum assay alone. However, patients with serum digoxin levels below 2.0 ng/ml are free of adverse effects, while those patients with serum levels above 2.7 ng/ml generally do manifest toxicity.

It is most important that the antiserum not recognize a difference between labeled and unlabeled antigen. If the antiserum were able to distinguish one from the other, the assay may be invalid. Many researchers, laboratory workers, and manufacturers have argued that the major alteration of the digoxin molecule with the addition of ^{125}I lessens the reliability of the assay. These people favor assays employing ^{3}H. However, in reality the assays, ^{3}H and ^{125}I, have been shown to have equal specificity and sensitivity. The reason for this apparent anomaly is the steroid specificity of the antiserum. Neither ^{125}I or ^{3}H alters the structure of the steroid portion of the digoxin molecule. There is growing enthusiasm over ^{125}I labeling because of interferences in liquid scintillation. For example, hemoglobin and bilirubin tend to quench fluorescence in liquid scintillation, hence lowering total counts. Some substances tend to fluoresce on their own, as is seen in the serum of patients with the uremia of kidney disease. It should be noted that uremic patients with cardiac difficulties are one of the primary groups in which blood digoxin levels are indicated.

Hepatitis B surface antigen

Principles. Acute viral hepatitis is a systemic disease primarily affecting the liver. There are two immunologically distinct forms of the hepatitis virus, type A and type B. The use of the terms "serum" and "infectious" hepatitis is frowned upon. Both type A and type B can be transmitted orally or parenterally. The hepatitis B virus (synonymous to serum or long-incubation virus) is a DNA virus that is capable of infecting the liver cells (hepatocytes). The core of the virus replicates in the hepatocyte nuclei. The virus surface material is synthesized in the

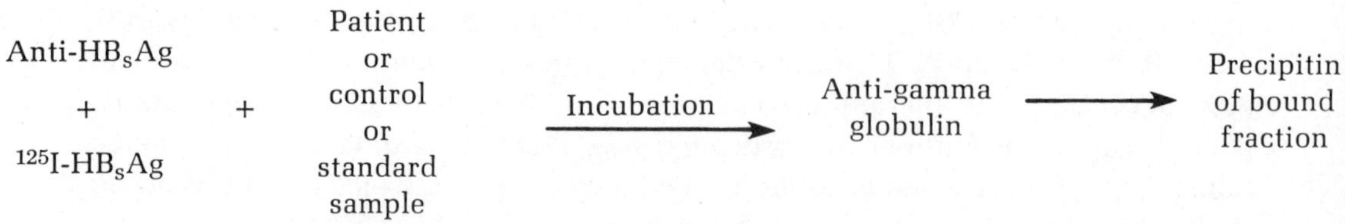

Fig. 9-19. Schematic representation of double antibody RIA for HB_sAg.

hepatocyte cytoplasm. This surface material is antigenic and is referred to as hepatitis B surface antigen (HB_sAg). During early infection excess HB_sAg is synthesized and released into the bloodstream. The HB_sAg is detectable by a variety of immunologic techniques. Later in the course of illness antibody to HB_sAg becomes detectable. Viral core antigens (HB_cAg) also are detectable in late infection.

Ovcr the past decade a series of assays have evolved to identify hepatitis-associated antigens. The earlier techniques such as agar diffusion or complement fixation assays were relatively insensitive. The newer techniques are by far more sensitive; accurate identification of hepatitis antigens is now possible. The most common use of the RIA for HB_sAg is in screening prospective blood donors for hepatitis.

Procedure. Double antibody or solid phase RIA techniques for detecting HB_sAg and anti-HB_sAg are commercially available. In the double antibody technique (Fig. 9-19) anti-HB_sAg is added to known concentrations of labeled HB_sAg (^{125}I-HB_sAg) and mixed with precise amounts of patient samples or controls. After incubation an anti-gamma globulin is used to precipitate the antibody-bound HB_sAg. This double antibody procedure separates the bound and free surface antigen. Centrifugation results in pelleting of the precipitate. Once centrifuged the free labeled HB_sAg is decanted and then the bound ^{125}I-HB_sAg is assessed for radioactivity in a crystal scintillation counter.

Interpretation. Presence of HB_sAg in a patient sample or a prospective blood donor's blood competitively inhibits binding of ^{125}I-HB_sAg to antiserum. This results in a decrease in isotope activity in the bound fraction and an increase in radioactivity in the free fraction. If HB_sAg is detected in the blood of a prospective donor, the person is not allowed to donate blood in an effort to reduce contagion. Identifying HB_sAg in a patient with hepatitis appears to be the only laboratory finding that distinguishes the type A hepatitis from the type B hepatitis.

Radioallergosorbent test (RAST)

Principles. The immunoglobulin IgE is known to be responsible for many allergic conditions as discussed in Chapter 2. Many attempts have been made to quantitate IgE levels by radial immunodiffusion and now by RIA. Interest in evaluating IgE blood levels has come from the physician in hopes that blood assays would aid in diagnosis and in evaluating treatment. However, a more important area of concern is identifying the offending allergens. Until recently, the only method available to identify the offending allergens in the allergic individual was skin testing. This process is somewhat cumbersome, unreliable, and often extremely uncomfortable for the patient. A new technique, however, provides the clinical laboratory with a means to identify the allergens and monitor changes in specific allergen IgE blood levels. This in vitro technique now known as RAST is based on the principles of RIA and is a major advance in the treatment and diagnosis of the allergic individual.

Procedure. Purified allergen, pollen or dander and so on, is coupled to inert particles forming an allergen particle complex (APC). Separate lots of APC are prepared for each allergen under study. The APC is then mixed with patient serum and incubated. During this incubation any antibody directed toward the particular complex allergen will bind to the APC. After incubation, the APC-antibody complex is washed with buffer. The mixture is then treated with ^{125}I-anti-IgE. The amount of isotope bound is directly correlated to the amount of patient IgE antibody to that particular allergen. In this way it is possible to quantitate the amount of IgE directed toward each allergen. This technique allows monitoring the changes in specific IgE antibody concentration with changes in therapy and life-style.

Interpretation. Retention of ^{125}I-labeled anti-IgE indicates the presence of allergen-specific IgE in the patient serum. By testing patient serum with different allergen complexes it is possible to screen patients for hypersensitivities to most of the common allergens. It is felt that effective treatment of allergies results in a decrease in IgE or an increase in allergen-specific IgG-blocking antibodies. By modifying the procedure one may use ^{125}I-anti-IgG to monitor changes in blocking antibody.

Homogeneous immunochemical techniques

Principles and limitations. Radioimmunoassays are heterogeneous techniques; the radioactive label is detected equally well in both the bound or free state. Because of this heterogeneity, it is necessary to separate the bound and free label. Imagine a technique in which the label is only active in the free form. This homogeneous technique would require no separation step. Labeled antigen bound to antibody would have no demonstrable activity; however, increasing concentrations of unlabeled antigen would compete for sites and free-labeled antigen. Once free, the label would then be active and measurable. It is not necessary to imagine such a system, for homogeneous assays already exist and are available commercially.

The sensitivity of labeled immunoassays is dependent on the affinity of the antiserum, the activity of the label, and the sensitivity of the detection systems. The homogeneous immunochemical techniques presently available are slightly less sensitive than the radioimmunoassay. However, these techniques offer some advantages. The major advantage is the elimination of the separation step, which is a source of error and is time consuming. Without a separation step the procedures are more easily automated, and it is likely the cost can be reduced substantially. There are two homogeneous immunochemical techniques presently available for clinical use; however, only one is presently suitable to the average clinical laboratory. The two methods currently available employ spin labeling and enzyme labeling. Most clinical laboratories are equipped with automated instruments capable of monitoring enzyme activity. For this reason most of the emphasis will be on enzyme immunoassay.

Enzyme-multiplied immunoassay technique

Principles and limitations. In the enzyme-multiplied immunoassay technique (EMIT, trademark of Syva, Palo Alto, California) enzyme is chemically bound to the antigen or hapten. The binding is thought to occur near the active site of the enzyme. Binding of antibody to the hapten (Fig. 9-20) blocks approximation and orientation of substrate to enzyme. In effect antibody binding to hapten sterically hinders substrate binding. Careful consideration of the above reaction reveals a curious and most useful phenomenon. Enzyme-hapten bound antibody has no activity, while the free hapten enzyme develops full enzymatic activity. This situation provides the laboratory with a system that is applicable to homogeneous immunotechnique.

In the homogeneous techniques the choice of enzyme to use in tagging to the hapten depends on several criteria. The enzyme must be readily available, easy to monitor, possess active grouping that may be used to link the enzyme to the hapten, have a high specific activity at a neutral pH, and must not be inhibited by substances present in biologic fluids. A commonly used enzyme in these assays is lysozyme. Lysozyme reacts with a substrate prepared from bacterial cell walls. The enzyme activity is monitored by a change in absorbance of the substrate while read in a spectrophotometer. High concentrations of free hapten in the controls, standards, or patient sample would tend to displace the enzyme-bound hapten from antibody. The greater the displacement of the enzyme-hapten complex the greater the enzyme activity and change in absorbance. Therefore there is a direct correlation between absorbance change and patient hapten concentration. The use of enzymes in immunoassays offers several distinct advantages over the use of isotopes: (1) the label is stable; (2) the activity is detectable without elaborate instrumentation; (3) the specific activity is high without a source of radiation danger; and (4) there is no need for a separation step.

EMIT—phenytoin

Principles. Phenytoin is an antiepileptic drug. This drug is an effective treatment for prevention of seizure activity in the epileptic patient. Like many drugs the benefits of therapy are obtained when the blood level of the drug is maintained within specific limits. Low blood levels are ineffective and high blood levels may be toxic. Accurate evaluation of phenytoin blood levels helps the clinician to maintain the patient at an effective, safe therapeutic dose. Blood levels reach a peak at 8 hours after the therapeutic dose and stabilize after approximately 3 days.

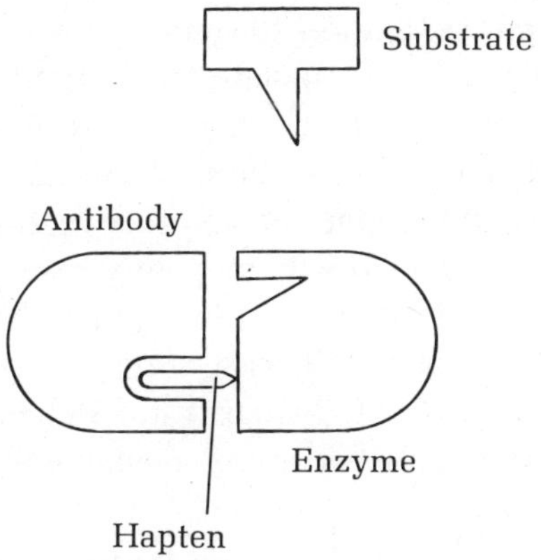

Fig. 9-20. In enzyme-multiplied immunoassays, hapten is coupled to enzyme somewhere in close proximity to enzyme's active site. Antibody binding to hapten blocks enzyme active site and inhibits catalytic activity of enzyme on substrate. Increased concentrations of free hapten in patient samples, controls, or standards react with antibody, allowing enzyme to react with substrate.

Procedure. The enzyme utilized in this assay is glucose-6-phosphate dehydrogenase (G-6-PD). The main reagent used in this test is a mixture of antiserum, G-6-PD-phenytoin, and substrate. As in RIA the antisera are diluted such that they are capable of binding 50% of the enzyme-linked hapten. In the first step of the assay, tubes are labeled for controls, patients, and standards. Reagent is dispensed into each tube. The appropriate samples (patients, controls, and standards) are added to their respective tubes. During an incubation time, patient drug competes for binding sites on antibody and displaces enzyme-linked hapten. Thus enzymatic activity increases with sample drug concentration. A high-patient or standard phenytoin level will bind most available binding sites, freeing the enzyme-linked phenytoin. The free enzyme-linked phenytoin, uninhibited by antibody, reacts with its substrate inducing detectable changes in absorbance. However, a patient with a low-phenytoin blood level would not be capable of displacing antibody-bound, enzyme-linked drug, and the result would be a very slow absorbance change in this assay. The enzyme utilizes nicotinamide-adenine dinucleotide (NAD) as a coenzyme (Fig. 9-21), and the NAD is reduced to $NADH_2$. The $NADH_2$ has a strong absorption peak at 340 nm. During the course of the enzyme reaction, the $NADH_2$ formed absorbs 340 nm. ultraviolet light, resulting in an increase in absorption. The rate of absorbance change at 340 nm. is proportional to the G-6-PD activity, which in turn is related to the phenytoin concentration in the patient sample.

Interpretation. Two absorbance readings, 30 seconds apart, are obtained at 340 nm on a spectrophotometer. The change in absorbance for five phenytoin standards, controls, and patient samples are then used to calculate the drug concentration. The 30-second absorbance change for the five standards is plotted versus their phenytoin concentration to generate a dose-response curve (Fig. 9-22). This curve is utilized to extrapolate the patient concentrations. The optimum therapeutic range is from 10 to 20 μg/ml serum. The serum levels vary depending on the time of last dose, the route of administration, the simultaneous use of other drugs, and individual metabolic variations. Severely hemolytic, lipemic, or icteric samples may result in poorly reproducible results. If drug assays are performed on urine, it is necessary to buffer the urine to optimize enzymatic activity. A variety of EMIT assays are commercially available (Table 23). At present, EMIT assays are primarily for detection and quantitation of drugs. However, the assay is now becoming available to measure metabolic sub-

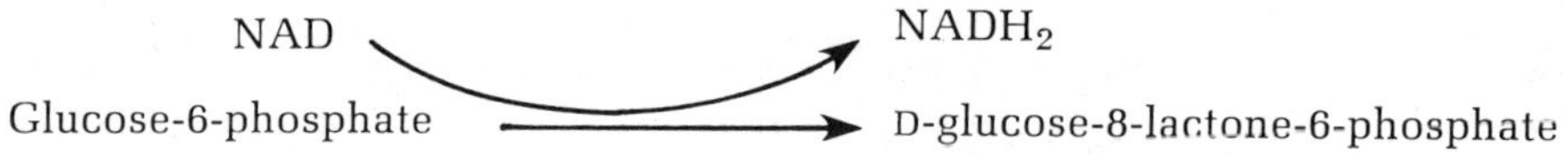

Fig. 9-21. Reaction utilizing G-6-PD in the phenytoin assay.

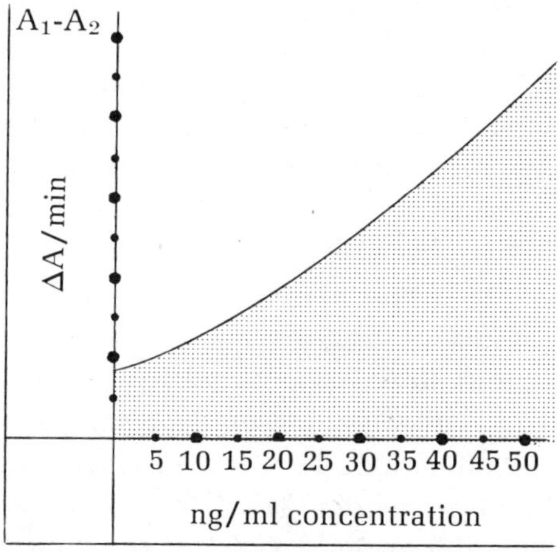

Fig. 9-22. Typical dose-response curve for serum phenytoin by enzyme-multiplied immunoassay. Change in absorbance, *A*, per minute is plotted versus drug concentration.

Table 23. Partial list of commercially available EMIT assays*

Drug abuse urine assays	Antiepileptic drugs	Cardioactive drugs
Opiate	Phenytoin	Digoxin
Amphetamine	Phenobarbital	
Barbiturate	Primidone	
Methadone	Carbamazepine	
Cocaine metabolite	Ethosuximide	
Benzodiazepine metabolite		
Propoxyphene		

*Syva. Co., Palo Alto, California.

stances such as thyroxine. An important bonus to the EMIT assay is that it can be modified to fit many types of automated chemistry instruments. Another major advantage of this assay is that it eliminates the need to handle radioactive material.

Electron spin immunoassays. An interesting modification of the EMIT is a system employing electron spin resonance spectroscopy (ESR). The electron spin spectrometer is an instrument capable of detecting molecules with unpaired electron spins by their characteristic behavior in an electromagnetic field. Unpaired electrons are relatively unusual in occurrence. For this reason antigen or hapten is labeled with a stable nitroxide radical (spin label). When the antigen–spin label complex is in the free form, it is detectable in an ESR spectrometer; however, in the antibody-bound form the nitroxide radical is unidentifiable. The spin-labeling characteristics provide all the makings for a homogeneous immunoassay similar to EMIT. Patient antigen and spin-labeled antigen compete for antibody-binding sites. The greater the concentration of antigen in the patient sample the more likely spin-labeled antigen will be displaced. When the tube containing the mixture is introduced into the ESR spectrometer, the signal generated will be proportional to the antigen concentration in the patient sample. The assay is commercially available for several drugs; however, there are some disadvantages to the technique, not the least being the scarcity of ESR spectrometers in the clinical laboratory.

Enzyme-linked immunosorbent assays (ELISA)

Principles. It appears that a new noncompetitive procedure known as enzyme-linked immunosorbent assays (ELISA) will be increasing in importance in the clinical laboratory. The ELISA technique can be used to detect antibody or antigen and employs many of the principles already discussed. Of crucial importance to the test is the fact that antigen or antibody can be bound to solid-phase medium and still retain immunoreactivity. The two principal techniques used are the double antibody technique for the detection of antigen and the indirect method for the detection of antibody. These assays have been used to identify a variety of infectious antigens, for example, viruses, fungi, and parasites as well as the antibodies these organisms may induce.

Double antibody sandwich ELISA. In the sandwich ELISA the solid phase material is coated with the specific antiserum, such as anti-HB$_s$Ag. The solid phase material can be a polystyrene microwell plate as used in the microserology systems. The sample being assayed for the suspected antigen is incubated in the antibody-coated wells. Thorough washing with buffer removes any unreacted material while antigen present is bound by solid phase antibody. The next step involves antibody specific for the trapped antigen. This second antibody is labeled with enzyme. Again a wash step removes any reacted conjugated antibody. The amount of enzyme bound is proportional to the amount of antigen in the specimen. The final step of the assay is to determine the amount of enzyme remaining in the well. This is accomplished by adding the enzyme's substrate and monitoring its activity. Depending on the enzyme substrate used, the assay may be read visually or quantitated by measuring activity in an optical system.

Indirect method. In the indirect ELISA one attempts to detect and/or quantitate antibody. Microplate wells are coated with antigen. The samples being assayed are added to the wells and incubated. Specific antibody present in the patient sample binds to the absorbed antigen and, in effect, is fixed to the microwell. Washing with buffer removes unreacted materials. Enzyme-labeled antihuman immunoglobulin is then used to mark the presence of specific patient antibody. Unbound enzyme-conjugated antibody is washed away with buffer, and the addition of substrate allows identification and quantitation of patient-specific antibody.

ELISA assays are not extensively used at the present time. The low cost of reagents, safety of the assay, reproducibility, sensitivity, and simplicity of the procedure will surely catapult the ELISA to a prominent position in the clinical laboratory in the near future.

READINGS AND RESOURCES

Aas, K., and Johansson, S. G. O.: The radioallergosorbent test in the in vitro diagnosis of multiple reagenic allergy, J. Allergy Clin. Immunol. **48:**134, 1971.

Ahluwalia, G. S., and Kuczala, Z. G.: Problems and evaluation of a ^{125}I-labeled digoxin radioimmunoassay relatively unaffected by hypoalbuminia, Lab. Med. **5:**29, 1977.

Ashkar, F. S.: Hepatitis and Australia antigen antibody studies, Lab. Med. **5:**30, 1974.

Avrameas, S., and Ternyek, T.: Peroxidase labeled antibody and FAB with enhanced intracellular penetration, Immunochemistry **8:** 1175, 1971.

Barrett, J. T.: Textbook of immunology, ed. 3, St. Louis, 1978, The C. V. Mosby Co.

Bastiani, R. J., Phillips, R. C., Schneider, R. C., and Ullman, E. F.: Homogeneous immunochemical drug assays, Am. J. Med. Technol. **39:**211, 1973.

Broughton, A., and Ross, D. L.: Drug screening by enzymatic immunoassay with centrifugal analyzer, Clin. Chem. **21:**188, 1975.

Catt, K., Niall, H. D., and Tregear, G. W.: Solid phase radioimmunoassay, Nature **312:**825, 1967.

Enquall, E., and Perlman, P.: Enzyme-Linked immunosorbant assay (ELISA). Quantitative assay of IgG, Immunochemistry **8:**871, 1971.

Freeman, L. M., and Blavfox, M. D., editors: Radioimmunoassay, New York, 1975, Grune & Stratton, Inc.

Goldman, M.: Fluorescent antibody methods, New York, 1968, Academic Press, Inc.

Hall, C.: Critical review of digoxin reagents and methodologies, Lab. Med. **5:**42, 1974.

Hollinger, F. B., Vordam, V., Smith, H., and Alter, H. J.: Assay of Australia antigen and antibody employing double antibody and solid phase radioimmunoassay techniques and comparison with passive hemmaglutination methods, J. Immunol. **107:**1099, 1971.

Howard, P. L., and Trainer, T. D.: Data handling and quality control in radioimmunoassay, Lab. Med. **5:**38, 1974.

Ishizaka, K., and Ishizaka, T.: Identification of E antibodies as carriers of reagenic activity, J. Immunol. **99:**1187, 1967.

Larson, S. M., and Thorell, J. I.: Principles of competitive radiobioassay, Lab. Med. **5:**15, 1974.

Leiva, B.: Separation techniques as guide in helping select an RIA kit, Am. J. Med. Technol. **43:**1, 1977.

Levte, R. K., Ullman, E. F., Goldstein, A., and Herzenberg, L.: Spin immunoassay technique of opiate narcotics in urine and saliva, J.A.M.A. **221:**1231, 1971.

Masaracchia, J.: Developing excellence in the performance of radioassays, Lab. Med. **5:**22, 1974.

Rabin, B. S.: Digoxin radioimmunoassay: clinical immunology. In Rose, N. R., and Friedman, H., editors: Manual of clinical immunology, Washington, D.C., 1976, ASM.

Rose, N., and Friedman, H., editors: Manual of clinical immunology, Washington, D.C., 1976, ASM.

Scharpe, S. L., Cooreman, W. M., Bloome, W. J., and Lee Keman, G. M.: Quantitative enzyme immunoassay, current status, Clin. Chem. **22:**733, 1976.

Skelley, D. S., Brown, L. P., and Besch, P. K.: Radioimmunoassay, Clin. Chem. **19:**146, 1973.

Stanworth, D. R.: IgE and hypersensitivity in man, Sci. Basis Med. 33-48, 1972.

Tietz, N., editor: Fundamentals of clinical chemistry, Philadelphia, 1976, W. B. Saunders Co.

Thomas, R. C.: Preparation of radioisotope labeled drugs, Annu. Rep. Med. Chem. **7:**296, 1972.

Yalow, R. S., and Berson, S. A.: Immunoassays of endogenous plasma insulin in man, J. Clin. Invest. **39:**1157, 1960.

Index

D

J

K

L

T